The ARTHRITIS Book

The ARTHRITIS Book

A Guide for Patients and Their Families

by
EPHRAIM P. ENGLEMAN, M.D.
and
MILTON SILVERMAN, PH.D.

with a foreword by
ROBERT J. GLASER, M.D.

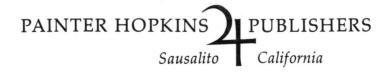
PAINTER HOPKINS PUBLISHERS
Sausalito *California*

Printed in the United States of America. Published
simultaneously in Canada by Clarke, Irwin & Company,
Limited, Toronto and Vancouver.

For information contact Painter Hopkins Publishers,
P.O. Box 1829, Sausalito, California 94965.

Library of Congress Cataloging in Publication Data

Engleman, Ephraim P.

    The arthritis book.
    Bibliography: p.
    1. Arthritis. I. Silverman, Milton Morris, 1910–
joint author. II. Title. [DNLM: 1. Arthritis—
Popular works. WE344 E58a]
RC933.E53   616.7'2   79-10470

ISBN 0-525-05850-8

1 2 3 4 5 6 7 8 9 10

To the arthritis patient

ARTHRITIS *is customarily defined as a state characterized by inflammation of one or more joints. Like many other definitions, this one is neither complete nor entirely accurate. In some forms of arthritis, there is little or no inflammation. In some, such as bursitis, it affects structures that are not strictly part of the joint. And in a few others, the disease may strike not only the joints, but also the kidneys, the lungs, the skin, the eyes, the blood vessels, or other parts of the body.*

CONTENTS

FOREWORD

The Arthritis Book is one of a series of short books by medical experts, written primarily but not exclusively for patients suffering from a given disease, in this instance arthritis in one form or another. I use the phrase *not exclusively* advisedly, because these books are also intended to be read by the families of patients. In the case of chronic afflictions such as arthritis, the patient's family and indeed his or her close associates are inevitably involved to some degree; they can contribute meaningfully to the patient's well-being.

Arthritis, the subject of this book, is an ancient disease, at least in some of its forms. Osteoarthritis, common in all of us as we grow old, has been known for centuries, and so too have forms of infectious arthritis. The remarkable progress in medicine recorded in this century, and particularly in the period since World War II, has resulted directly in the recognition of new or hitherto unrecognized forms of arthritis. In some instances the disease may simply have been undetected in an earlier time; in others, diseases with significant arthritic components may well represent the unexpected consequences—the paradox—of progress. Here I refer especially to a disease such as disseminated lupus erythematosis (see Chapter 6), which may result in some instances from untoward bodily reactions to new drugs.

Most chronic illnesses, certainly, are identified with discomfort, disability, or deformity. Arthritis, however, brings all three. Fortunately, as the authors of this book properly point out, we have come to understand much more about many forms of arthritis, and have made great strides in easing the burden borne by arthritis sufferers. For example, those forms of arthritis associated with bacterial diseases such as gonorrhea, meningococcal meningitis, and tuberculosis are now readily treatable once the diagnosis is established or even seriously suspected. Prior to the advent of the sulfonamides and the antibiotics, all of these forms of arthritis usually produced joint destruction and ultimate crippling. In some instances, with disease progression, death was the ultimate outcome. Today, prompt treatment obviates complications and almost always ensures a favorable outcome.

In other forms of disease such as rheumatoid arthritis, treatment methods have improved gratifyingly, and overall support of the patient has increased his or her ability to carry on a satisfying, productive life.

Moreover, just as the progress to which I referred earlier has brought the advances discussed in this book, continuing research, utilizing sophisticated scientific methods, holds promise of even more effective methods of early diagnosis and prompt treatment.

Frequently a patient and his or her family has little or no understanding of the particular disease with which he or she is afflicted. Often persons without understanding lack appreciation of the whys and wherefores of treatment and the long-term outlook. Physicians being extremely busy people cannot always give patients detailed information and full explanations of their problems. This book is designed to complement the physician's role by providing an authentic, objective description of the various forms of arthritis and their treatment. The text is prepared for the layman, in language that does not presuppose a scientific background on the part of the reader. This book does not take the physician's place; rather, it puts repeated emphasis on the patient's responsibility to follow the regimen prescribed by the doctor. Answers to many questions may be found here, but, if they are not, the patient should seek them from the physician. It is particularly important that the patient adhere carefully to the physician's treatment instructions and never alter the medication plan unless the physician concurs. Self-medication is frequently the pathway to trouble.

A word about the authors, whose friendship and collaboration dates back to their undergraduate days at Stanford, is in order. Each is well recognized in his respective field.

Dr. Ephraim P. Engleman was graduated from the Columbia University College of Physicians and Surgeons in 1937, and had his clinical training in medicine at the Mt. Zion and University of California hospitals in San Francisco and at the Pratt Diagnostic Hospital in Boston. After a fellowship at the Massachusetts General Hospital under Dr. Walter Bauer, an acknowledged leader in applying a sophisticated scientific approach to the study of arthritis, Dr. Engleman entered the Army Medical Corps and served as chief of the rheumatic fever center at the Torney General Hospital. Since 1946, Dr. Engleman has been a member of the faculty of the School of Medicine, University of California, San Francisco, where in 1965 he was made clinical professor of medicine and chief of the arthritis clinics at the medical center. He has served as a member of many important committees and study groups concerned with arthritis, and in 1975–76 had the distinction of being chairman of the National Commission on Arthritis and Related Musculoskeletal Diseases, established by the National Arthritis Act, PL-93-640. He is currently director of the Rosalind Russell Medical Research Center for Arthritis, a member of the National Arthritis Advisory Board, and president-elect of the International League Against Rheumatism.

Dr. Engleman was one of the first rheumatologists to investigate the use of cortisone in the treatment of rheumatoid arthritis, soon after Hench, Kendall, and their associates demonstrated the dramatic effects of this steroid hormone. He has continued to evaluate new forms of therapy in various types of arthritic disease, and has published more than a hundred papers as well as a number of chapters in medical textbooks dealing with arthritis.

Dr. Engleman is a warm, compassionate physician, devoted to his patients, and dedicated to the continued development of improved diagnosis and better treatment of patients with arthritis. He is also a gifted teacher.

Milton Silverman, Dr. Engleman's co-author, received his Ph.D. in 1938 in biological sciences from Stanford University. For twenty-five years he was science editor of the *San Francisco Chronicle*. He also wrote extensively on science for a number of national publications including the *Saturday Evening Post, Colliers,* and the *Reader's Digest,* among others. He is a past president of the National Association of Science Writers, and a winner of a Lasker Award for distinguished medical reporting.

The author of a number of books about drugs, including *Pills, Profits, and Politics,* which he wrote in collaboration with Dr. Philip R. Lee, former Assistant Secretary for Health and Scientific Affairs in the Department of Health, Education, and Welfare, Dr. Silverman was executive secretary of the HEW Task Force on Prescription Drugs and has been a consultant to various other governmental bodies. He is now a member of the senior faculty of the Health Policy Program, University of California San Francisco Medical Center, and a lecturer in pharmacology in the schools of medicine and pharmacy.

April, 1979   Robert J. Glaser, M.D.
                                      Consulting Professor of Medicine,
                                      formerly Vice President of
                                      Medical Affairs and
                                      Dean of the School of Medicine,
                                      Stanford University

ACKNOWLEDGMENTS

We are deeply indebted for the invaluable help provided by our clinical and scientific colleagues in preparing and reviewing this book, and by the many patients who gave generously of their time and thought in telling us what questions *they* wanted to have answered. None of them, of course, bears any responsibility for our statements.

Our particular gratitude goes to the following:

HOWARD POLLEY, M.D., of the Mayo Clinic

LAWRENCE SHULMAN, M.D., and DONALD WHEDON, M.D., and their co-workers of the National Center of Arthritis, Metabolism, and Digestive Diseases, and many members of the National Arthritis Advisory Board

ROBERT GILBERT, M.D., of Children's Hospital, the Shriner's Hospital for Crippled Children, and the University of California in San Francisco

MARTIN SHEARN, M.D., of the Kaiser-Permanente Hospital, Oakland, California

EDGAR ENGLEMAN, M.D., of Stanford University

ARTHUR CERF, M.D., of Mount Zion Hospital, San Francisco

CLYDE HOCKETT, M.D., of the family practice programs at the Yakima Valley Memorial Hospital and St. Elizabeth's Hospital, Yakima, Washington

CHARLES BENNETT and his colleagues of the Arthritis Foundation in Atlanta

DOROTHY RICE, THOMAS HODGSON, and their associates in the National Center for Health Statistics

JAMES RUSSO, formerly of the Pharmaceutical Manufacturers Association and now of Smith Kline & French, and officials of the manufacturers of the major anti-inflammatory drugs

RALPH SCHAFFARZICK, M.D., of Blue Shield of California

ELLIOTT WARSHAUER and the many other San Francisco area pharmacists who opened their pricing files to us

ACKNOWLEDGMENTS Our colleagues DAVID BULLARD, KRISTINE ROMINGER, SANDRA LEWIS, KENNETH SACK, M.D., DONALD BESTE, RICHARD deLEON, WALLACE EPSTEIN, M.D., and PHILIP R. LEE, M.D., of the School of Medicine and the School of Pharmacy, University of California, San Francisco

For devotion far beyond the call of duty, JEAN ENGLEMAN and MIA LYDECKER

And, for the inspiration she kindled in all of us who knew and worked with her on the National Commission on Arthritis, the dedicated, gallant, and utterly charming ROSALIND RUSSELL

January, 1979   Ephraim P. Engelman, M.D.

Milton Silverman, Ph.D.

The ARTHRITIS Book

CHAPTER 1

SCOPE OF
THE PROBLEM

Wе live in a world of rising expectations and hold to the optimistic belief that medical research and health-care delivery will continue to improve the lot of human beings. Most of us have high hopes of longer, healthier lives for ourselves and our children. In the case of arthritis, the future looks promising.

In the past few decades, there have been encouraging advances in the understanding and treatment of this age-old disease. These advances are improving the care given arthritis patients by physicians, both rheumatologists, who specialize in arthritis, and general practitioners and internists. Increasingly, physicians are able to make accurate diagnoses and select the best treatment for the particular patient and the form of the disease.

This book is written not only for patients suffering from arthritis, but for their families and friends as well. Much new information is presented. There are ample grounds for a positive viewpoint. Arthritis need not lead inexorably to deformity and pain. Its complications are rarely fatal. Some diagnostic and therapeutic procedures are so new that many patients and even some physicians may be unaware of them. A well-informed patient will seek the right kind of professional advice early—and not after years of delay—and will follow that advice intelligently.

In the United States today, arthritis is generally considered to be the most widespread, crippling, disabling, and often most painful of all the chronic illnesses. In many ways it is the most baffling, more baffling even than such others as asthma, heart disease, high blood pressure, and chronic kidney disease. For most forms of arthritis, no cause has yet been identified. In an individual patient, it is difficult if not impossible to predict if or how the disease will progress.

Arthritis is not a single disease but a large group of

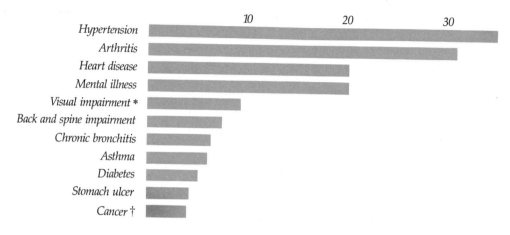

PREVALENCE OF SELECTED CHRONIC DISEASES *(In millions of patients)*

SOURCES: 1978 approximations from the National Center for Health Statistics; National Heart, Lung, and Blood Institute; National Cancer Institute; Arthritis Foundation; American Cancer Society; and National Institute of Arthritis, Metabolism, and Digestive Diseases.
* Impairments not correctable by glasses.
† Nonmelanoma skin cancers not included.

conditions. For the sake of simplicity, the various forms considered here will be lumped together under the name arthritis, rather than the more technical and cumbersome phrases "arthritis and related musculoskeletal disorders" or "rheumatism and rheumatic diseases" that some physicians prefer.

In the United States, arthritis is becoming increasingly prevalent. In part, this is a consequence of the success of medical research and clinical practice in controlling other diseases. Most serious infectious ailments have been brought under control by sulfa-drugs or antibiotics. Fewer newborn babies die, fewer mothers perish in childbirth, and fewer adults are killed by pneumonia, tuberculosis, meningitis, typhoid fever, and other dreaded infections of the past. As a result, more people survive to reach middle and old age, the years in which they are most likely to be afflicted by most forms of arthritis and other chronic illnesses.

Thirty-one million people in the United States alone suffer from arthritis—one out of every seven Americans. More than sixteen million of them have osteoarthritis, six

4

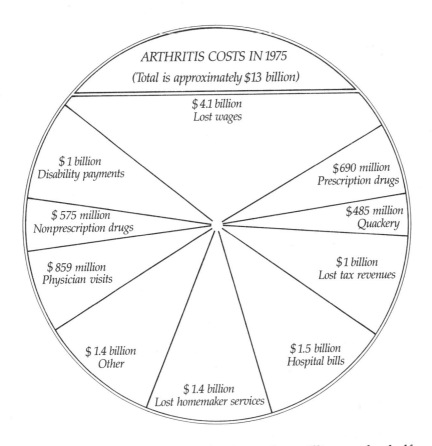

ARTHRITIS COSTS IN 1975
(Total is approximately $13 billion)

$4.1 billion
Lost wages

$1 billion
Disability payments

$690 million
Prescription drugs

$575 million
Nonprescription drugs

$485 million
Quackery

$859 million
Physician visits

$1 billion
Lost tax revenues

$1.4 billion
Other

$1.5 billion
Hospital bills

$1.4 billion
Lost homemaker services

million have rheumatoid arthritis, and a million and a half have gout. Some studies show that more than 90 percent of people over sixty years of age have at least a sign of arthritis that can be detected by x-ray examination, yet most are essentially symptom-free. Both men and women suffer from arthritic diseases, but most forms are more prevalent among women. And people with low incomes and from rural areas are more likely to be afflicted than are those with high incomes and from cities. It is mainly a disease of the elderly, but it may strike children. Today the prevalence of arthritis among children is higher than that of polio during the most severe epidemics of the past.

The financial costs of the disease to patients, insurance companies, health plans, and taxpayers are staggering. The price Americans paid in 1975 was more than thirteen billion dollars. One and a half billion went for hospital care, and almost a billion more for consultation with physicians. About three-quarters of a billion dollars was spent on prescription drugs, and more than a half billion on nonprescription drugs: unfortunately, an additional half billion dollars was squandered on charlatans and quack remedies. More than four billion dollars was lost in wages that would otherwise have been earned, and a billion dollars was lost in tax revenues. At least a billion dollars was spent on disability payments, and almost one and a half billion was lost in homemaker's services. In 1978, the combination of an increase in the number of arthritis patients, the use of more expensive treatments, and inflation resulted in an expenditure estimated at twenty-five billion dollars.

It is obvious that arthritis will place an increasing financial burden on society. Rising costs, increasing longevity, and the delivery of health care to a growing percentage of the population will combine with people's rising expectations to make the treatment of arthritis an even greater concern to all. As alarming as these financial costs may be, they are easier to understand than the physical and emotional costs to the patients and their families. As one patient put it, "How do you figure the cost of a lifetime of frustration?"

The treatment of many forms of arthritis is largely dependent on the use of drugs. The most common is aspirin, not in the small doses used for a headache, but in much larger amounts. In addition, many prescription drugs have been tested and approved for use under a physician's supervision. The selection of such drugs requires a physician's knowledge. There must be concern for the frequency and amount of the medication, and careful and informed observation of both beneficial effects and possible side effects. But drugs alone are not enough. One of the greatest positive factors in the successful treatment of arthritis depends on how well the patients are motivated to participate in their treatment, noting any changes in their symptoms, observing their own reactions to medication; recognizing their own fears or hopes or worries, and communicating all such information frankly and accurately to their physicians.

It cannot be stressed too strongly that early diagnosis can help to minimize later pain and disability. Arthritis treatment is a fight for time. Early treatment and careful, faithful compliance with the physician's advice will give the patient a far better chance for arresting, alleviating, or, in some cases, actually curing the disease. The newer drugs, described later in this book, have helped many, as have increasingly successful surgical procedures. Everyone af-

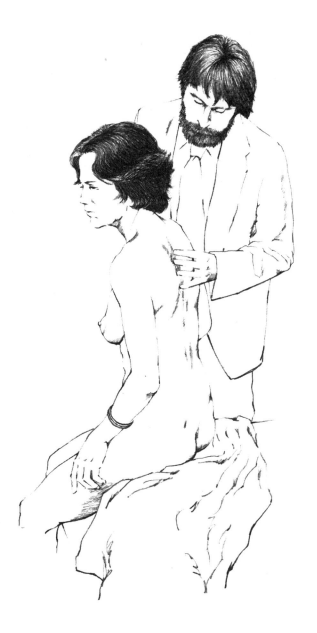

fected directly or indirectly by arthritis has much to gain in
this fight for time. New and improved drugs will almost
surely continue to become available. Physicians and other
professionals will become increasingly skillful and knowledgeable in applying individual and team treatment. The
number of medical specialists in the field will continue to
grow, as will the number of special medical facilities needed
for those with severe arthritis problems.

7

Research on the many complex factors that may affect the onset and the control of arthritis is a promising and exciting field. A few forms of arthritis, it is known, are caused by bacterial or viral infection, and other infectious agents may eventually be incriminated. Recently it has been realized that most forms of arthritis may result from the malfunction of the body's own defensive immune system. It is thought that this system, which normally acts to reject foreign material—a microbe or a splinter, for example—from the body, may fail to recognize the difference between the body's normal components and the foreign invader; the resulting inflammatory reaction may be responsible for the damage in the joints. Much more needs to be understood about genetic factors that may play a role, and many research laboratories are engaged in experiments along these lines. Many major hospitals now include immunological units in their clinical laboratories; they help physicians determine which patients are most at risk, reach an accurate diagnosis, and prescribe appropriate treatment.

There are between eighty and a hundred distinct varieties of arthritis. Some are quite similar to each other, while others appear to be totally different. Some forms attack joints and the tendons and muscles associated with joints. Some strike not only joints, but such organs as the kidneys, lungs, skin, eyes, blood vessels, and even the brain. In some patients, for no known reason, the symptoms disappear for months or years, only to recur. In some cases, the disease disappears permanently. Certainly the situation is not bleak.

Some forms of arthritis whose complications once led to death can now be effectively controlled with drugs.

Only a few years ago, an uncommon form of arthritis known as systemic lupus erythematosus was rapidly fatal; only about 50 percent of its victims survived as long as five years after diagnosis. Now 90 percent survive ten years or longer.

Another once highly destructive form, infectious arthritis, is now quickly controlled and usually cured by modern antibiotics.

Although millions of patients have rheumatoid arthritis, one of the most serious forms of the disease, many have only occasional bouts of discomfort, lasting only several weeks or perhaps a few months. Many live with little or no inconvenience or pain, are not disabled, remain employable, and are free to lead active lives.

Another form of arthritis, gout, was once associated with extreme pain and physical deformity. Formerly and mistakenly thought to be a disease resulting from "gluttony, boozing, and wenching," gout is now readily controllable. Serious complications are virtually unknown.

For some forms of arthritis, the use of heat and cold treatments, braces, and specially designed exercises usually provides substantial relief.

More and more sufferers are receiving help—often dramatic help—from new forms of surgery. Effective operations are performed to insert plastic or metal substitutes for damaged joints. For example, total hip replacement, surely one of the impressive advances of modern surgery, now has a success rate of approximately 95 percent and is performed on about eighty thousand people each year in the United States. It has brought new lives to many older people, some in their eighties and nineties. Other procedures mend torn tendons, reshape deformed fingers and toes, and restore motion to "frozen" joints.

For most patients, whether they are fighting their first skirmishes with the symptoms of arthritis, or whether they find themselves face-to-face with advanced disease, the most critical question may be this: How does one go about finding the best advice? It is important to turn to a well-trained physician who has an interest in arthritis, is up-to-date, and is both knowledgeable and sympathetic. In most cases, the physician need not be an arthritis specialist. Excellent care can be provided by many general practitioners or family physicians, internists, and pediatricians. There is no need for most patients to flock to university or teaching hospitals and medical centers. This is fortunate, because there simply are not enough specialists and specialized clinics. In the United States, with thirty-one million people with arthritis, there are three thousand rheumatologists. Although at least a quarter of million children have arthritis, there are only a small number of pediatricians trained in its treatment. Among orthopedic surgeons, there are relatively few who have had special training and experience required for the surgical reconstruction or replacement of damaged joints.

A patient should seek out the right physician and follow his advice. But there are a few physicians who are clearly not fitted by training or temperament to deal with arthritis. A physician who states that the case is "hopeless" or dismisses the problem with a remark that the patient is merely getting old should be left for one with understanding and sympathy. Effective medical care demands mutual respect and even friendship between physician and patient. In the treatment of no disease is this more true than in arthritis.

Experts generally agree that treatment should start early in the course of the disease. Unfortunately, estimates indicate that 75 percent of arthritis victims postpone seeking medical care for four years or more after their first symptoms appear. Thus, part of the arthritis problem lies in these delays in seeking medical help.

Although most cases of arthritis can be treated satisfactorily by physicians who are not specialists, this is not always the case. Patients, along with their physicians, families, and colleagues, should be aware of those signals that indicate the time has come to call for special help from a rheumatologist, an orthopedic surgeon, or a special care unit. What are these warning signals?

Indications that the disease is affecting an increased number of joints, or that it is involving such organs as the heart, lungs, or skin, for instance.

Signs of increasing deformity in the joints, motion becoming more limited and painful, muscles weakening, increasing fatigue, loss of weight and appetite, or fever.

Indications that the disease has progressed to the stage at which aspirin and other relatively nonhazardous drugs are no longer effective and therefore that more potent but more hazardous agents such as gold salts and hormones like cortisone may be needed.

Signs that surgery may be needed to alleviate pain and disability.

Seriously increasing depression or other significant emotional problems.

Most cases of arthritis are relatively easy for a physician to diagnose and treat. In others, however, there may be great difficulty. Even with the most sophisticated diagnostic services available and consultation with colleagues, it may take months to arrive at the proper diagnosis. It may be equally baffling to find an effective treatment program. But we have complete confidence in the remark made by a physician recently:

I've never seen an arthritis patient I couldn't help.

CHAPTER 2

SCENE OF THE CRIME

Arthritis was an old disease long before the first caveman killed his first saber-toothed tiger and the first cavewoman learned how to use fire. It afflicted dinosaurs and flying reptiles more than a hundred million years ago. It probably appeared along with the development of the spine and has plagued four- and two-legged vertebrates ever since.

Today it affects not only human beings, but also elephants, rhinoceri, hippopotami, horses, cattle, hogs, dogs, cats, chickens, turkeys, rats, and mice. (*Mice?* Absolutely. One of the best experimental animals for the study of one form of arthritis is a strain of New Zealand mice.)

In most forms of arthritis—the word comes from the Greek *arthron*, or joint, and *-itis*, meaning inflammation—the joint is the chief scene of the crime.

According to an old song, the ankle bone is connected to the shin bone, the shin bone is connected to the knee bone, the knee bone is connected to the thigh bone, and so on. This may be marvelous material for a barbershop quartet, but not for accurate anatomy. In fact, in most animal joints, bone is not connected to bone. Rather, the end of each bone is covered with a smooth, glistening, living tissue called gristle, or cartilage. In the typical joint, the cartilage covering the end of one bone moves smoothly over the cartilage covering the end of another bone, almost without friction.

This bone-cartilage–cartilage-bone arrangement is encased in a relatively soft tissue called the joint capsule. The inner lining of the capsule is known as the *synovial membrane*. Filling the joint space and lubricating the cartilage is the *synovial fluid*. What goes on in the synovial membrane, the synovial fluid, and the cartilage may not mean the difference between life and death to an arthritis patient, but it may mean the difference between comfort and agony.

13

The capsule does not isolate an individual joint from the rest of the body. Running through the capsule and its inner lining is a network of tiny blood vessels that, among other things, carry nourishment to the joint structure. These small blood vessels may also bring in bacteria, fungi, viruses, destructive chemicals, helpful drugs, and perhaps other factors that may either induce arthritis or control it.

Also running through the capsule and the synovial membrane are nerves, including those that conduct sensations of pain to the brain.

Around the joint are various soft tissues—muscles, tendons, and ligaments—that are technically not part of the joint but can be involved in the arthritis process. They can be weakened, atrophied, torn, or otherwise damaged.

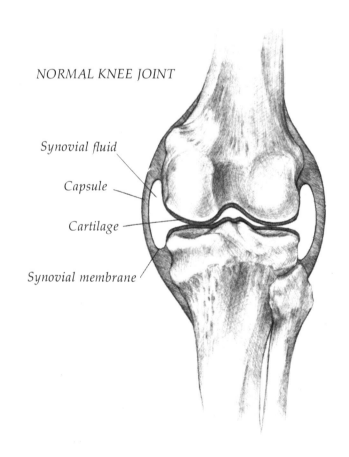

NORMAL KNEE JOINT

Synovial fluid

Capsule

Cartilage

Synovial membrane

This whole joint structure may not be perfect. Perhaps modern engineers could have designed it better and more foolproof. But this is the design that human beings have inherited, a design that has served us reasonably well for many millions of years. Until a better design is introduced, this is the one that most of us will have to live with. Or suffer with.

CHAPTER 3

RHEUMATOID ARTHRITIS

[The Misery-All-Over Disease]

Of the common forms of arthritis, the one probably least desirable to have is rheumatoid arthritis. Second only to osteoarthritis—the so-called wear-and-tear arthritis—in prevalence, it afflicts about six million people, with a ratio of roughly three women to one man.

Rheumatoid arthritis is characterized by inflammation, with joints that are painful, stiff, swollen, warm, and tender, and sometimes by deformity and crippling. Generally, the onset is insidious, with pain and slight inflammation in perhaps a few joints in the hands or feet. Later, it may migrate, striking other, larger joints—such as the wrists, knees, elbows, ankles, and hips. Almost always the condition is symmetrical, involving, for example, both hands or both knees.

There may be stiffness and pain, especially in the morning after a patient has been nearly motionless all night, that may last for an hour or two or longer. The stiffness may recur in the course of the day after either prolonged sitting or excessive exercise.

In many patients the disease may produce what have been described as sick-all-over or misery-all-over symptoms. Often there is loss of appetite, weight loss, fatigue, weakness, and low-grade fever. Rarely does it attack the lungs, heart, eyes, nerves, or blood vessels.

In some patients, it may be found that the first manifestation of the condition came after a physically stressful situation, such as an acute infection or physical injury. In others, it was preceded by severe emotional stress, such as with separation, divorce, or the death of a close friend or relative. Occasionally, the condition seems to be related to continuing emotional tension or stress at home or on the job. Most often, no such precipitating factor can be found. Stress, however, can trigger a new flare-up of the disease.

Unlike wear-and-tear arthritis, which becomes increasingly evident in middle-aged and elderly people, rheumatoid arthritis may begin at any age but does so most commonly between the ages of twenty and forty. Sometimes it progresses remorselessly, with more joints seriously involved. There can be periods in which the symptoms are especially severe and others marked by substantial or complete relief. In some cases, the disease seems to burn itself out, and the patient may be symptom-free from then on.

It is of great importance to understand that proper treatment—especially if it is started early in the course of the illness—can usually control pain and minimize joint deformity, crippling, and disability. Among expert clinicians, there seems to be agreement that at least 75 percent of the patients who start appropriate treatment early in the disease—those having had symptoms for less than twelve months—will show substantial improvement, and from 15 to 20 percent may be completely relieved of symptoms. Even though there may be obvious stiffness, pain, or limitation of motion, 50 percent or more of the patients are still able to take care of themselves and are fully employable ten years later. Some reports indicate that, from ten to fifteen years after the onset of the disease, from 50 to 70 percent can hold fulltime jobs, and only about 10 percent are completely disabled.

In rheumatoid arthritis from the outset, there is the mystifying, severe inflammation and overgrowth of the synovial membrane, the inner lining of the joint capsule. As the disease progresses, there is destruction of the cartilage and the underlying bone, along with changes in the surrounding muscles and other soft tissues that can lead to pulling one bone out of alignment with another, resulting in joint deformity. As a joint becomes increasingly damaged, there may be moderate to severe pain that can limit motion. On the other hand, many people with gnarled, misshapened fingers have no significant pain and can effectively perform as typists or do knitting or embroidery.

What sets off this devastating inflammation remains a major mystery. Early workers were convinced that it is caused by an infection—and some modern investigators still suspect that it may be. In some respects, it acts like an infectious disease. There is clear evidence that infection can, indeed, lead to rheumatoidlike disease in cattle, sheep, swine,

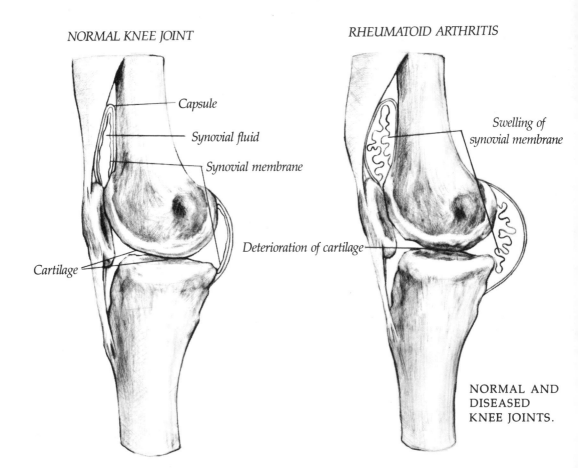

NORMAL KNEE JOINT

Capsule

Synovial fluid

Synovial membrane

Cartilage

RHEUMATOID ARTHRITIS

Swelling of
synovial membrane

Deterioration of cartilage

NORMAL AND
DISEASED
KNEE JOINTS.

and rats. But in human beings, there is yet no convincing evidence that bacteria, viruses, or other microorganisms are implicated.

As far as heredity is concerned, there appears to be no evidence that rheumatoid arthritis runs in families. In fact, it is not unusual to find that, when one of a pair of identical twins is afflicted, the other is not.

Some workers seem to feel that the disease is another result of various pollutants in the modern environment, but scientists believe that rheumatoid arthritis is as old as the creation of bones and joints. Epidemiologists have reported that the incidence of the disease may vary in different parts of the world, or in different parts of the United States, but no consistent pattern has shown up to offer a useful explanation.

From the knowledge that we have today, what seems to be involved is a strange immune process in which the body

21

turns against itself. Normally, inflammation is considered to be a good thing rather than a bad thing. It is usually a part of the body's defensive tactics to protect its tissues against foreign invaders, living or dead. The invader may be a pneumococcus organism (which causes pneumonia), a typhoid bacillus, the toxin produced by a diphtheria organism, or a polio virus. All such invaders—or some chemicals contained in them—are called *antigens*. Ordinarily, they stimulate the body to produce *antibodies*—for example, an antipneumococcus antibody, an antityphoid antibody, an antidiphtheria toxin antibody, or an antipolio antibody. Unfortunately, the terms antigen and antibody cannot be defined both simply and completely; the situation is reminiscent of that in which a monk is described as a man who lives in a monastery, and a monastery is defined as a place in which monks live.

In recent years, the antigen-antibody immune reaction has played a critical role in organ transplants—for instance, the transplant of a kidney or a heart from one person to another. The transplanted tissue is likely to be rejected as a foreign body unless the host's immune mechanism is temporarily dampened with immunosuppressive drugs. (As will be noted later, such suppressive drugs are now being tested in arthritis treatment.)

In rheumatoid arthritis, a similar antigen-antibody mechanism seems to be functioning, but the antigen—the substance that triggers the immune response—has not yet been found. It may be an infective bacterium or virus, or possibly a substance produced by the body itself, but no identification has yet been made. Regardless, the antigen-antibody complex in rheumatoid arthritis turns against the body's own tissues—the synovial lining of the joint, the cartilage, and the bone. In complicated cases, the lungs, heart, blood vessels, and other tissues are attacked as if they were foreign invaders.

The diagnosis of this kind of misdirected internal warfare is often easy, based on simple examination of the patient. Sometimes it is far more complex, and the physician may have difficulty in distinguishing rheumatoid from other types of arthritis and, accordingly, in deciding on the best treatment.

In diagnosis, a careful and complete history and physical examination are essential. X-ray examinations and labo-

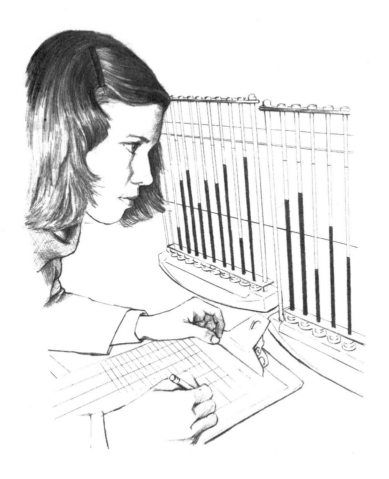

MEASURING THE
SEDIMENTATION
RATE.

ratory tests can be helpful. Measurement of the sedimentation rate—determining how rapidly red blood cells sink in a glass tube—is valuable as an indicator of any kind of inflammation. One simple, relatively rapid, and inexpensive technique is a blood test for the presence of a peculiar protein called *rheumatoid factor*. This factor is present in most patients with rheumatoid arthritis but not in all of them. Further, it is present in some perfectly healthy subjects. Presence or absence of rheumatoid factor must be considered only a possible diagnostic aid.

In taking the patient's history and planning a course of treatment, the prudent physician will ask questions like these:

When did the symptoms first appear? Which joints were involved first? Were the first symptoms preceded by any physical or

23

emotional stress? Did it happen after a bout of influenza or dysentery, or after you worked in the garden, or after a divorce or a death in the family?

Is there anything like this in your family? (Certain forms of arthritis seem to be inherited.)

In the first attack, how long did the symptoms last?

Did you take any medicine? Did it help? Or did it make you feel worse? (Certain patients are allergic to particular drugs or cannot tolerate them.)

What drugs are you now taking for arthritis or for anything else? Has any drug ever made you ill? (Some antiarthritis drugs may interact with other medications. Sensitivity to a nonarthritis drug may carry over to an arthritis remedy.)

Are your attacks associated with a sudden increase in temperature? (A "yes" answer may indicate the presence of infectious arthritis and the urgent need for antibiotics.)

Are your attacks marked by excruciating pain in the big toe? (A "yes" answer may indicate gouty arthritis, again with a different form of therapy.)

Is your body weight normal, high, or low? What is your usual diet? (Proper body weight and a balanced diet are recommended for everyone.)

Is your problem the aching knee, or hip, or wrist, or is it really the fact that the sore joint makes it impossible to knit, or crochet, or type, or have customary sexual relations, or go bowling with your friends, or deal a bridge hand?

When you awaken in the morning, do you feel sore and stiff for five minutes? Twenty minutes? An hour? Two hours? (Prolonged stiffness may, for example, be present in rheumatoid arthritis but not in osteoarthritis.)

What is your financial status? How much health insurance coverage do you have, and what does it cover? Will it cover office visits, x-rays, laboratory tests, hospitalization, surgery, and both in-hospital and out-of-hospital drugs? Under your Medicare, Blue Shield/Blue Cross or other policy, there may be a deductible requirement that you must meet by out-of-pocket payment.

How compatible are you with the people with whom you live— your spouse, a companion, children?

From what you have heard or read about arthritis, what do you think or fear or *know* will happen to you? (Some patients are convinced that their problem will always remain of minor importance, while others are certain that they cannot be helped.)

Have you been impressed by articles that you have read or reports that you have heard about arthritis patients who have been dramatically helped (or grievously harmed) by super doses of

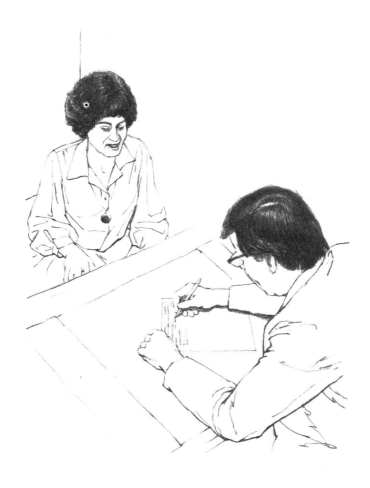

Vitamin C or Vitamin E or Vitamin B-complex, by diets of wheat germ or bean sprouts, by acupuncture, hypnosis, daily enemas, biofeedback, by rubbing counterirritant (and usually smelly) ointments over the painful joints, by moving to Nepal? (Interestingly, any of these procedures may make some patients feel better for brief periods, but unfortunately there is no evidence that any one of them has a measurable effect on the progress of the disease.)

Which of your hobbies are becoming difficult or impossible because of arthritis? What hobbies do you have—playing the violin, stamp collecting, reading, photography—that are still comfortable and emotionally rewarding?

How high (or how low) is your tolerance for pain? (The answer may well influence the choice of treatment.)

If a patient's symptoms are already disabling, the physician may ask in addition:

What are your living arrangements? Do you live alone or with somebody else? Can that person help you physically and emotionally? Are helpful friends, relatives, or neighbors available?

What does your job require of you? Does it consist of heavy physical labor? How dependent are you on your job? Can you cut down to halftime, or quartertime, at least temporarily? Can you change jobs?

Is your home or apartment all on one floor? Must you use stairs? Or is an elevator available?

Are there children in the family? How many and how old? How dependent are they on you, physically, emotionally, and financially?

Not all such information is necessary for the treatment of every patient. Further, not all of the questions can be asked and answered in the ten or so minutes available in an average office visit. But, for a rheumatoid arthritis patient with clearly progressing disease, more pain and increasing crippling, these questions must be asked and answered. For such patients, it is vital that the physician and the patient develop as early as possible a relationship of mutual understanding and trust. To develop such rapport, competent physicians will often schedule at least one 1-hour session (and perhaps more) to obtain information that may eventually be critical to the care of the patient.

After rheumatoid arthritis has been diagnosed, even tentatively, a program of treatment must be designed specifically for that patient. The elements of such a program may include balanced rest and exercise, the application of heat or cold or both, the employment of specially shaped braces or other supports, dietary restrictions (primarily to reduce excess weight), drugs, and surgical repair. An integral part of such a program is the willingness of both patient and physician to discuss all aspects of the problem frankly. It is also important for the patient to disregard recommendations from well-meaning friends, neighbors, and relatives to ignore the prescribed treatment.

In most cases, for the best long-term outlook, conservative management is far better than aggressive or more spectacular approaches. Aggressive methods may sometimes have dramatic results, but too often they cause side effects that can range from annoying to catastrophic.

The conservative treatment for rheumatoid arthritis is, up to a point, much like that for many other forms of arthritis.

Patients must be protected wherever possible from physical and emotional stress, fatigue, and other factors that may precipitate a rheumatoid bout or aggravate the existing condition. They should not attempt to undertake spring housecleaning all in one day, or to weed the entire garden after it has been untended all winter. Where possible, they should avoid occupations with tight deadlines. They should be advised not to participate in any type of work or sport in which further injury to a joint is likely.

Avoiding situations that may further damage an arthritic joint is only one part of the program. Taking time to rest—from 30 to 60 minutes twice a day—is usually helpful.

For some patients, warm compresses applied for a few minutes several times daily will combat pain and inflammation. Others seem to get more relief from cold compresses.

Because patients often feel stiffness and pain when they awaken, a warm (not hot) bath or shower for 5 or 10 minutes may be recommended. This is most effective if taken immediately after getting out of bed.

Mild forms of exercise, individually designed for each patient, are essential. They should be performed for a few minutes several times every day. A vigorous, three-hour workout once a week is not an appropriate substitute. Nor is jogging, long-distance running, or the like. Such activities may be excellent for strengthening muscles, and building morale, but they may only further damage already affected joints. Above all, exercising to the point of exhaustion or increasing pain should be avoided. As one physician puts it, "If you have more pain after nine holes of golf, don't play eighteen."

Some patients have reported that they feel better after staying at a health resort or spa, or moving to a warm, dry climate. It is certain that these feelings are common, but there is no evidence that such a climate has any effect on the progression of the disease. This matter will be discussed further in the next chapter.

Often, splints or braces worn only at night or for a few hours each day can be helpful. These are not the heavy metal

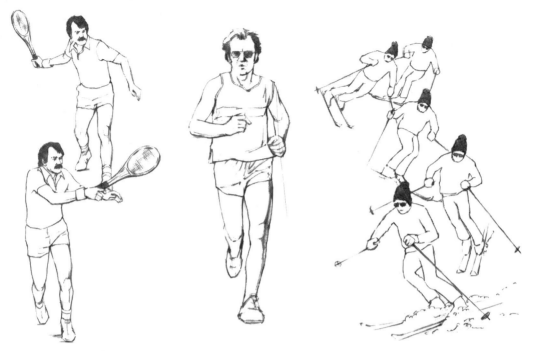

VIGOROUS EXERCISE MAY FURTHER DAMAGE JOINTS
AFFECTED BY RHEUMATOID ARTHRITIS.

or plaster casts used in the past, but lightweight metal or plastic devices. They can be purchased from stock, or they can be ordered to fit a particular joint in a particular patient. They can be prescribed either to support a weight-bearing joint or to keep such joints as those in the fingers, hand, or wrist in the proper position overnight.

Most expert rheumatologists seem to agree that the overwhelming majority of rheumatoid arthritis patients can obtain relief of symptoms from the use of anti-inflammatory drugs. Treatment may be needed for weeks, often for months, sometimes for years. The drug initially prescribed is usually aspirin, the daily dosage being restricted by a patient's tolerance of the drug—that is, just below the point at which such adverse reactions as stomach distress or ringing in the ears occur.

As will be noted in a later chapter, there is a multitude of aspirin products on the market, many of them available at strikingly different retail prices.* Providing the dosages and

* For a further discussion of aspirin and other antiarthritis drugs, see Chapter 11.

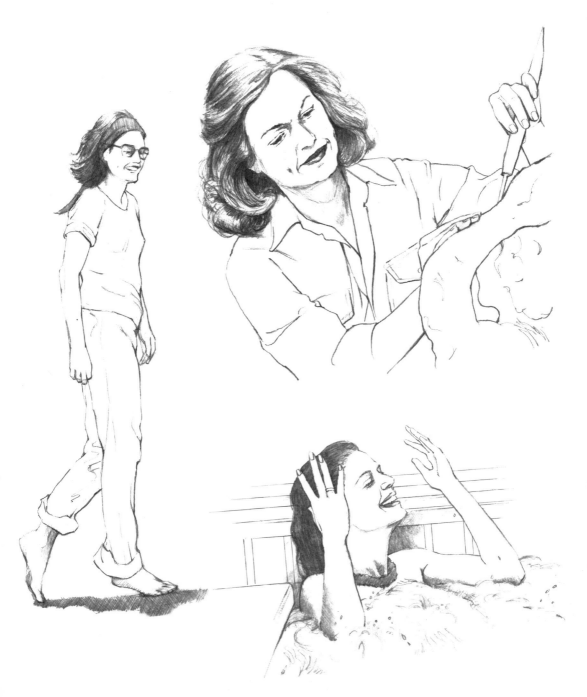

MILD EXERCISE, RELAXATION, AND WARM BATHS ARE BENEFICIAL.

aspirin content are the same, their effects on the rheumatoid process are essentially identical.

Also available are an exceedingly large number of combinations of aspirin with other drugs. There are drugs that may be useful for alleviating headache or fever but have no antiarthritis value; nonetheless they are promoted for the treatment of "the minor pains of arthritis."

Besides aspirin are other agents classified as nonsteroidal anti-inflammatory drugs—that is, like aspirin in proper doses, they help to control inflammation. Among them are such substances as phenylbutazone, indomethacin, and hydroxychloroquine, the last originally introduced for malaria treatment. More recent additions include fenoprofen, ibuprofen, naproxen, tolmetin, and sulindac. In a different class are such agents as gold salts and penicillamine. Their use is marked by greater hazards, and consultation is usually recommended.

Finally there are the corticosteroid hormones such as cortisone and its derivatives. They may be injected directly into an acutely painful joint or taken orally if several joints are involved. The latter route of administration can have dramatic effects in reducing inflammation, pain, stiffness, and disability. Moreover, they often produce a sense of euphoria, and the sensation of resting on a cloud. But the potential adverse side effects of this entire family of hormones are—or should be—all too well known to physicians. Caution is indicated, and consultation may be desirable.

The decision to resort to gold salts or to the oral use of steroids or penicillamine means that conservative therapy is no longer adequate, and that more radical measures can no longer be postponed. This decision is generally based on many factors. Despite conservative therapy, the disease is progressing and becoming out of control. Motion of the affected joints is becoming increasingly restricted. There is more stiffness, joint deformity, and pain. Other joints are being affected. There are signs that the disease is producing change in other organs. There is more fatigue, more constant low-grade fever. And the patient is losing interest in family, friends, vocation, and hobbies.

To make the best decision, the family physician and a consultant—usually a rheumatologist—should share their knowledge. In some cases, it may be decided that the patient should be hospitalized for a week or two to enable the physician to make a better appraisal of the situation. How does the patient actually perform the recommended exercises? Can personal instruction from a physical therapist help teach the patient or a family member how to do the exercises correctly? Are new x-ray examinations or laboratory tests desirable? What happens to the patient's emotions and morale when family members are not always present?

Another approach is surgery. While anti-inflammatory drugs are administered to suppress inflammation and physical therapy and exercise are prescribed to maintain joint function and muscle tone, surgery is utilized to alleviate pain or improve function in a joint that has already been seriously damaged. Operations range from the simple procedure of removing inflamed tissues from the lining of an affected joint to such massive procedures as total replacement of an entire hip or knee. At this point, knowledgeable family physicians and internists, who usually take care of most patients with mild to moderate arthritis, will invariably refer the patient to an orthopedic surgeon.

In this general attack against rheumatoid arthritis, it seems desirable to consider a team approach*—and to consider it long before all elements will be needed. Consultation may be sought with physical therapists, social workers, vocational rehabilitation experts, and other professionals. If surgery is needed, the family physician or rheumatologist will call for consultation with an orthopedic surgeon substantially ahead of the time that surgery may be scheduled.

Family members, other relatives, and friends should be urged to take part in this team effort. In particular, wives, husbands, and children should be made aware of the physical and emotional factors that may become important or critical. They should know that there will probably be up-and-down periods, and the patient may desperately need emotional support when the disease flares up. Since most patients are women, help from family members may be necessary to ease the burdens of cooking, cleaning, bedmaking, and caring for children.

When necessary, a patient's employer should be included in the team and be informed of the possible course of the disease and the possible need for limitation of employment, fewer working hours each day, or a job change. Often,

* See Chapter 15.

if given enough warning, a thoughtful employer can find a different and less strenuous job for an employee, rather than discharging him.

Obviously, the cost of treatment must be considered. There must be careful examination of the insurance coverage of a patient facing serious medical or disability problems. It must be recognized that hospitalization alone, at average costs ranging now from $150 to $200 per day, can amount to $2,000 or more, surgical expenses can run from $1,500 to $15,000 or more, and even out-of-hospital drugs (not now covered under Medicare) can cost as much as $100 a month.

In summary, although the exact cause of rheumatoid arthritis remains unknown and no cure has yet been discovered, early diagnosis of the disease and the prompt initiation of treatment—including the advice of experts at appropriate times—can minimize or prevent crippling in most cases. Moreover, with the application of new medical, surgical, and rehabilitative methods, even those who have been seriously disabled can be restored to an active and productive life.

So, what does a person suffering from rheumatoid arthritis do? Get the best medical advice possible and follow it. Carry adequate health insurance. And don't quit.

A few years ago, the National Commission on Arthritis reported to the Congress the case of a 27-year-old attorney, three years out of law school, who developed the first sign of rheumatoid arthritis. At the end of two years, he was barely able to work. Then, after the use of antiarthritis drugs, surgical operations on both knees, and other treatments carefully supervised for years by expert rheumatologists—years in which the attorney and his wife subsisted mainly on Social Security disability and welfare payments—the disease was slowly brought under control. At the end of three years, he was able to start law practice again on a part-time basis, and finally, ten years after his arthritis began, as a full-time attorney—and taxpayer.

It had been, the patient noted, a long ten years.

But he didn't quit.

CHAPTER 4

OSTEOARTHRITIS
[The Wear-and-Tear Disease]

Unquestionably the most widespread form of arthritis is that known as osteoarthritis, often called wear-and-tear arthritis or the arthritis of old age. Somewhat more common in women than in men, it is relatively rare in those below the age of thirty-five. It can be detected by x-ray examination in 87 percent of women and 78 percent of men over the age of sixty-four. It obviously affected dinosaurs, cavemen, and Egyptian pharoahs. If, as the Bible relates, Methuselah lived to the age of nine hundred sixty-nine, the wear-and-tear ailment probably made life miserable for him, but this has not been thoroughly investigated by biblical scholars.

Unlike other, more serious forms, osteoarthritis is generally marked by relatively little inflammation, and relatively little serious deformity. The lungs, heart, kidney, eyes, or other organs are not affected and relatively few joints are involved. There is no fever, no loss of appetite, no sick-all-over feeling.

According to x-ray studies, an estimated 40 to 50 million adults in the United States have signs of the disease, but many may not be aware of it. X-ray photographs may reveal that many of an individual's joints have been affected, but the person is essentially symptom-free and not to be categorized as a patient.

The striking lack of correlation between what the x-rays show and what the patient feels has long puzzled experts. With practically identical joint changes, as disclosed by x-ray examination, a few victims may be seriously incapacitated, but most can carry on their customary household duties, hold their usual jobs, play golf, ski, jog, and cavort with their children or grandchildren.

In the case of the primary form of osteoarthritis, there is no apparent explanation for the start of the disease. For some reason, probably related to hereditary factors, changes occur in certain complicated protein-carbohydrate substances in the cartilage. Over years—probably many years—the cartilage shows signs of cracks like those that appear in old marble. Later these cracks become deep fissures, and the cartilage is ulcerated, eroded, and destroyed. As the end result of these changes, there may be a compensatory overgrowth of bony tissue in the joint, which becomes enlarged, painful, and stiff. Or there may be no discomfort at all. The joint is rarely red, hot, or inflamed.*

In secondary or traumatic osteoarthritis, usually limited to one or two joints, the cause seems to be related to injury—resulting, for instance, from a congenital defect, a fracture, or an automobile or sports accident. Ordinarily, it takes years after such an insult to the joint before the osteoarthritis becomes apparent. The condition may also be brought on by years of overweight, bad posture, or occupational overuse of a particular joint.

Primary osteoarthritis comes on slowly and usually hits the small joints at the ends of the fingers and then one or more of the weight-bearing joints. In the finger joints, hard but usually painless lumps—known as Heberden's nodes—may develop. Their presence often helps physicians diagnose the disease.

Traumatic osteoarthritis most frequently involves the hips, knees, and ankles. Shoulders, knees, and hips are notably affected in those who participate in football, basketball, soccer, and other contact sports. Some authorities have commented on the involvement of the fingers in typists, pianists, and baseball players, the ankles in ballet dancers, the thumb in gardeners, and the wrists in golfers and operators of pneumatic drills. A particularly painful variety, probably related to faulty alignment of the lower jaw, can affect joints connecting the jaw to the skull. Others have noted that a cause-and-effect relationship may be nonexistent, and emphasize that many typists and pianists do not have arthritic fingers, and many professional football players—well, at least some of them—have healthy hips and knees.

* Osteoarthritis of the spine, a somewhat different form, is considered in the following chapter.

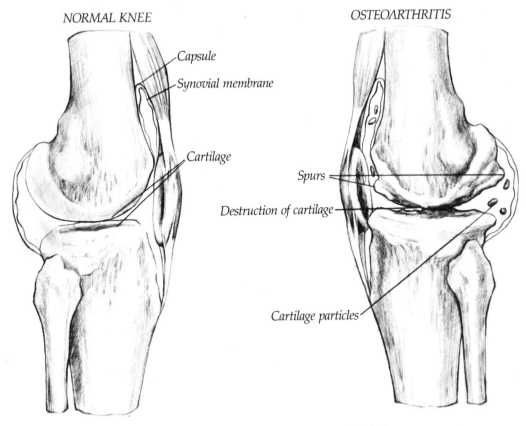

NORMAL KNEE

Capsule

Synovial membrane

Cartilage

OSTEOARTHRITIS

Spurs

Destruction of cartilage

Cartilage particles

NORMAL AND DISEASED KNEE JOINTS.

Whether a relationship exists between trauma and a particular case of arthritis has frequently been a matter of controversy in medical-legal disputes in which, for example, a plaintiff may sue for arthritic damages allegedly resulting from an automobile or industrial injury that occurred at some time in the past.

There appears to be no doubt, however, that wear-and-tear arthritis occurs more frequently in those engaged in heavy physical labor.

Regardless of how and where the disease starts, the cartilage destruction and overgrowth of bone proceeds in the same manner, but to a totally unpredictable degree. In the majority of cases, the disease progresses to the point at which there is slight or moderate pain on effort—which is alleviated by rest—and slight stiffness, especially for a few

37

minutes on arising. The stiffness may also be evident after sitting too long in one position. There may be some limitation of motion. This limitation may be totally unimportant to most people, but it can be disastrous to a seamstress, for example, or a violinist. It is only infrequent that the condition progresses still further, to serious deformity, crippling, and severe pain.

In osteoarthritis, the degree of pain is of strategic importance. It can range from annoying to incapacitating; in addition, severe pain can make it almost impossible to exercise the joint.

With this form of disease, physicians rarely need to worry about suppressing inflammation, since it seldom occurs and then is usually mild. The primary goal of treatment is simple—*control the pain.*

Occasionally the pain and stiffness will disappear spontaneously, with or without treatment, and the patient will be well for weeks or months. But if treatment is needed, the program is built on a combination of approaches: adequate but not excessive rest; a reducing diet for patients who are overweight; local heat applied through use of warm compresses or a warm (not hot) bath immediately on getting out of bed; mild rather than vigorous exercise; and the use of drugs. Regular physical therapy is usually not needed or worth the expense. Where drugs are concerned, the modern physician has a remarkable selection of agents for use. Despite the minimal amount of inflammation in most patients, anti-inflammatory drugs often provide considerable symptomatic relief. Unquestionably, aspirin remains the first drug of choice, usually taken with meals or with an antacid. For those who obtain no help from large amounts of aspirin or for the relatively few who cannot take it without gastric distress or other unpleasant side effects, other products are available. Among these are indomethacin and such newer substances as fenoprofen, ibuprofen, naproxen, tolmetin, and sulindac. All are more expensive than aspirin and may or may not be more effective.

In osteoarthritis, cortisone-like hormones are sometimes injected directly into a particularly painful joint but are not ordinarily given by mouth.*

* For a more detailed description of these and other antiarthritis drugs, their generic and brand names, and their relative costs at the retail level, see Chapter 11.

For centuries, it has been fashionable for those who could afford it to spend many weeks or months at a health spa, or to move to a warm, dry climate. Under such conditions, many arthritis patients—regardless of the type of their disease—unquestionably feel better. Neither the spa atmosphere nor the warm, dry climate, however, has a detectable effect on the course of the disease. The warm baths of a spa may be helpful to relieve symptoms, but they are no better than warm baths in the privacy of one's own bathroom. The mineral waters, which are supposed to be ingested in large quantities, are ineffective. A warm, dry climate may provide relaxation and emotional tranquility for those whose lives are normally full of tension, but it might be noted that natives of Florida, New Mexico, Arizona, and Southern California also are victims of arthritis.

Those contemplating a more or less permanent move should consider carefully the financial and emotional factors—giving up a job, finding new living accommodations and perhaps a new life-style, and leaving family and friends. In some cases, of course, getting away from irritating family members and neighbors may be just what the doctor would suggest.

The standard basic treatment—rest, heat, and drug therapy—does not exhaust the possibilities. Where needed, lightweight plastic casts can be used to provide temporary support for a painful joint. Canes and crutches can help a patient walk without discomfort. Of growing importance is the use of surgery.

In most cases of osteoarthritis, the primary, and perhaps the best, reason for turning to the surgeon is for relief from pain—not so much to repair a deformed joint, or one that is limited in range of motion, as to control extreme pain that cannot be overcome safely by the use of any drug treatment. If a patient is no longer able to rest at night and to perform essential tasks, surgery deserves careful consideration.

Depending on the joint involved and the type and amount of cartilage destruction and bony overgrowth, there are perhaps a dozen different surgical procedures that may be considered, ranging from the fusion of two bones that are painful on movement or reshaping the end of one bone or another to the total replacement of the entire joint with a metallic, ceramic, or plastic substitute.*

* For a description of the main surgical procedures used in arthritis, see Chapter 12.

Probably the most satisfactory results—and certainly the most dramatic—have come with total replacement of the hip. This is a major procedure often taking two to three hours or more and usually requiring from two to three weeks of hospitalization. With modern methods of anesthesia, the use of antibiotics to prevent or control postsurgical infection, and other improvements, it has become remarkably safe. In this country alone, hip replacement is performed on tens of thousands of patients each year. In most cases, pain is almost completely controlled, motion is almost entirely restored, and the patient can return to normal activity.

CHAPTER 5

ARTHRITIS
IN THE SPINE

Many thoughtful anatomists have agreed that whoever designed the spine—that remarkable structure including bony vertebrae, discs, muscles, and nerves—did not contemplate the possibility that vertebrate animals would ever do anything but walk on four legs. It seems all too clear now that the human spine was never designed for a species walking on two legs. Two-legged ambulation clearly produces stresses and strains with which the spine is not constructed to cope.

The result of this modern insult to an outmoded structure is only too evident. It is marked by what patients describe variously as spinal arthritis or spinal rheumatism, usually but not always involving either the lower back or the neck or both. Regardless of what patients may label it, arthritis in the spine represents a major challenge to orthopedists and orthopedic surgeons, who claim that it accounts for as much as 40 percent of the problems which afflict their patients. Often, the diagnosis is not clear in the early stages.

From the symptoms described by the patient, it is not always easy to determine whether the problem represents mainly a muscular spasm or other disorder, primarily joint disease in the vertebrae, or some complex combination of muscle and joint problems.

In this chapter, attention will be focused on two major spinal diseases—noninflammatory osteoarthritis of the spine and an inflammatory condition bearing the jaw-breaking name of ankylosing spondylitis, commonly called poker spine, ramrod spine, or frozen spine.

Spinal Osteoarthritis

A major cause of the "Oh, my aching back!" syndrome, spinal osteoarthritis commonly but not invariably accompanies advancing age. In many respects, it is similar to osteoarthritis of the fingers, toes, knees, and hips. Usually it is marked by little or no inflammation. Instead, there is destruction of the vertebral joint cartilage, followed by overgrowth of the bone, including the growth of bony spurs that are detectable by x-ray examination.

In the spine, these bony overgrowths can sometimes produce seemingly unrelated symptoms. If such a spur impinges on nerves running to or from the hands or feet, for example, the symptoms may include numbness and tingling in the fingers or toes.

Ordinarily, the older the patient, the more there is cartilage destruction and bony overgrowth. There is, however, no necessary relation between symptoms and x-ray findings. There may be massive changes in the bony structure and yet the patient may have no significant symptoms, while there

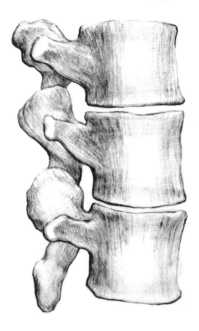

NORMAL VERTEBRAE

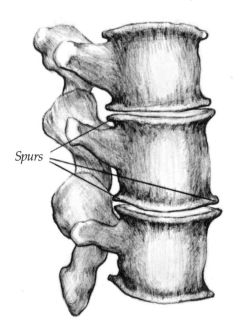

VERTEBRAE WITH SPURS

Spurs

may be only minimal changes detectable by x-rays and yet the patient suffers from severe back pain and disability. Moreover, the symptoms may be caused by a condition other than arthritis.

Treatment of spinal osteoarthritis is basically the same as that for other kinds of osteoarthritis—rest, a carefully designed program of daily exercise, applications of heat or cold, and administration of aspirin or such other antiarthritis drugs as indomethacin and the newer nonhormonal anti-inflammatory substances. Even though inflammation is minimal, as is the case with osteoarthritis in general, these anti-inflammatory agents may produce excellent results. Some patients may benefit substantially from weight reduction.

In some instances, traction—such as stretching the upper part of the spine, in the region of the neck—may be recommended and used cautiously under supervision. The value of such traction is not clear. Some physicians believe it has merit. Others are not convinced. There seems to be more evidence that a patient can get at least temporary relief by using a neck collar or simply a towel wrapped around the neck. There is no evidence, however, that use of either traction or a collar influences the progression of the illness.

The "Stiff Spine"

Ankylosing spondylitis (meaning "stiff spine") is a painful and sometimes crippling inflammatory condition vastly different from osteoarthritis of the spine. It usually appears in young adults, especially young men between the ages of twenty and thirty. Unlike osteoarthritis, which is essentially a noninflammatory disease of the joints, it is an inflammatory disease, with complications that may involve the eyes, the heart, and, rarely, the lungs. Roughly one-quarter of the patients suffer an eye complication, which usually can be easily and quickly detected and controlled, but which may lead to permanent eye damage or blindness if left untreated.

While osteoarthritis may start in the upper or lower parts of the spine, ankylosing spondylitis almost always begins in the lower portion of the back, particularly the sacroiliac joints. It is occasionally accompanied by shooting

45

pains in the thighs that at first may resemble the pains of sciatica. Early in the disease, there may be few physical signs to explain the symptoms. Patients may be dismissed as malingerers, or told they are using their backs as outlets for a neurosis or other emotional problem. The condition may be misdiagnosed as a totally different arthritic or muscle disorder. As the disease worsens, it seems to march upward in the spine, either afflicting each higher vertebra in turn or skipping one or two and then attacking the next.

Infrequently, in advanced cases, the spine becomes increasingly stiffened or frozen in position. This may result in a spine that is as stiff and straight as a poker or ramrod. Even less frequently, it is immobilized in the shape of a curve, and the patient may find it virtually impossible to lift his head to a normal position in order to see, and he is forced to walk with his chin practically resting on his chest. In many cases, these changes may be prevented by early treatment.

Also in advanced cases, the disease affects the spinal joints to which the ribs are connected. Normal rib motion becomes painful, as in pleurisy, and the victim breathes not by chest motion but by raising and lowering the diaphragm. Chest expansion may be completely inhibited, and the patient seems to inhale and exhale by means of his abdomen. This, too, can probably be prevented by early treatment.

Since 1973, it has been known that diagnosis of ankylosing spondylitis can be aided by the detection of a particular antigen or a genetic marker known as HLA B-27 (HLA stands for *human leucocyte antigen*). Early workers in the field of immunology believed that this marker was attached only to leucocytes, or white blood cells. During the past few years, it has been found attached to a variety of other cells in the body. From 6 to 9 percent of normal, healthy white subjects possess the genetic marker; thus, occurrence of the marker does not necessarily show that the disease is present. In contrast, in white patients with true ankylosing spondylitis, it occurs in 90 to 95 percent. The antigen is not commonly found in healthy black individuals, and the disease is uncommon among blacks. The results of recent studies suggest that the condition exists in more women than was previously believed, but usually in a mild form.

In approximately 50 percent of the patients, there may be transient involvement of such other joints as the hip or shoulder. In about 25 percent, however, this joint involvement may be permanent. The involvement of other joints

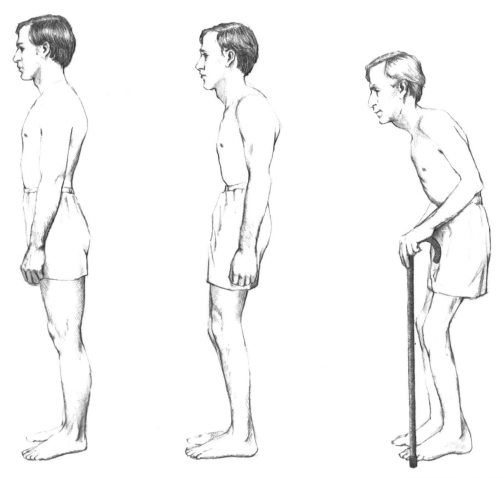

PROGRESSIVE CHANGES IN ANKYLOSING SPONDYLITIS OVER TWENTY YEARS. [AFTER *ARTHRITIS AND ALLIED CONDITIONS: A TEXTBOOK OF RHEUMATOLOGY,* 8TH ED. J.L. HOLLANDER AND D.J. MCCARTY, JR., EDS. LEA & FEBIGER, 1972.]

such as the knees may mimic rheumatoid arthritis. In the latter condition, however, a blood test can usually detect the presence of "rheumatoid factor," which is rarely present in the spinal disease. Furthermore, rheumatoid arthritis rarely affects the low back. Ankylosing spondylitis should be suspected in any young man or woman complaining of chronic back pain.

Effective treatment of the disease is based on the usual antiarthritis program: rest, exercise, the use of warm baths or showers, and the administration of anti-inflammatory drugs, beginning with aspirin. Gold salts and hydroxychloroquine are ineffective, and the need for corticosteroid hormones is rare. Phenylbutazone and indomethacin are

47

probably the most effective, but it would seem that the newer nonhormonal anti-inflammatory agents are also useful.

Where there has been severe deformity of the spine, surgical procedures have been employed, sometimes with excellent results. The surgery, however, may be accompanied by serious risks of causing further spinal injury, nerve damage, or rupture of major blood vessels, which must be explained in full to any potential candidate for the operation.

Although the results of delayed or inadequate treatment once seemed to make ankylosing spondylitis one of the most devastating forms of arthritis, modern diagnosis makes it actually one of the easiest to detect in relatively early stages, and modern methods of treatment can bring it under more or less complete control.

The essential part of modern treatment is a course of simple exercises that must be performed faithfully several times a day and can be done easily at home. These exercises

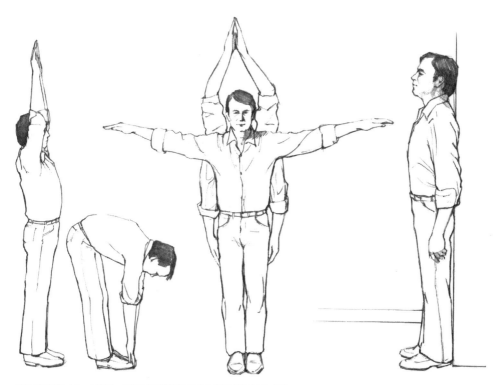

POSTURAL AND BREATHING EXERCISES FOR ANKYLOSING SPONDYLITIS.

are neither vigorous nor dramatic. They are aimed at developing and maintaining proper posture and proper breathing. Sleeping on a firm mattress is desirable, along with the use of a small pillow or none at all. Swimming is often helpful. In this disease, perhaps the greatest value of anti-inflammatory drugs is to permit exercise with a minimum of pain.

Patients have to realize that they must stay on this do-it-yourself routine for the rest of their lives. Each patient must learn again how to sit, stand, and walk. If this lesson is learned, most patients will be able to function normally, hold almost any kind of job, and live essentially normal lives.

For what was once such an ominous disease, this is not a bad ending.

CHAPTER 6

LUPUS

[*The Great Masquerader*]

Of the diseases with arthritic manifestations, systemic lupus erythematosus (SLE, or lupus) can be one of the most serious. Frustrating to the patients and their families who must live with it, and exasperating to physicians and researchers who attempt to diagnose, treat, and understand it, the disease is probably more prevalent than cystic fibrosis or muscular dystrophy or multiple sclerosis. Yet, it seems, few patients have ever heard of it until they themselves are told that they have it. Few doctors have had extensive experience in dealing with the disease.

Recognized by physicians as a specific disease only since about 1900, lupus was once thought to be almost inevitably fatal. As recently as the 1940s, only one patient in six survived as long as three years after diagnosis. Now most of them are able to live reasonably normal lives most of the time, and the death rate has been slashed dramatically.

What had long baffled physicians in coping with the disease was the bizarre, kaleidoscopic set of symptoms that may occur in lupus. Not all of them strike the same victim, but usually several of them appear together. There may be a butterfly-shaped, reddish rash across the bridge of the nose, extending to one or both cheeks, or on the chest, so that many patients first consult a dermatologist or allergist. There may be swelling in the joints, which may be misdiagnosed and mistreated as rheumatoid arthritis. In lupus, these joint changes usually do not cause deformities. Often fever, malaise, lack of appetite, and weight loss will be noted. There may be signs of anemia, or bleeding from the nose or vagina. There may be peculiar mental changes that will seem to call first for psychiatric care. The hair may fall out. There may be signs or symptoms suggesting chest disease, heart disease, abdominal disease, or kidney disease. The patient may go from one specialist to another before the true diagnosis becomes obvious enough to indicate the proper course of treatment.

A deranged immune reaction or reactions, possibly to some unidentified infectious agent, seems to be responsible for this mystifying condition. There is one male to about seven or eight female victims in the white population. It is three times more common in blacks than in whites. The number of victims in the United States is estimated to be between 100,000 and 200,000 or more. It usually appears in patients between the ages of fifteen and thirty-four. It may run in families.

To the patients themselves, perhaps the most unhappy symptoms are those stemming from the effect of lupus on the brain. These central nervous system changes may range from mild or subtle to striking, and from depression to mania. There may be epileptic-like convulsions. Tremendous strains are placed on friends and family members who want to offer help but do not know what form that help should take. Often the patient feels lonely, angry, misunderstood, and totally helpless. .

Today this disease, with its sometimes awesome array of symptoms, can usually be controlled and reversed. First, however, a diagnosis must be reached. Sometimes this is far from a simple procedure, and it may take three or four months or longer for the disease to progress to the point at which the diagnosis can be made.

Modern lupus diagnosis generally requires a careful medical history and a battery of studies. For example, the symptoms may be caused by a number of different drugs that the patient is already taking for diseases unrelated to arthritis. These must be ruled out. Depending on the individual case, the physician will probably order various blood tests, urine tests, x-rays of the joints, studies of lung and heart function, and even skin or kidney biopsy, or measurement of brain waves. Ordinarily the blood tests are designed to measure the sedimentation rate of red blood cells and detect what are known as antinuclear antibodies and LE (for lupus erythematosus) cells, serum complement, and anti-DNA antibody. These measurements are essential not only for confirming or excluding lupus, but also for telling how the disease is progressing, whether the treatment is working, and when a flare-up might be expected.

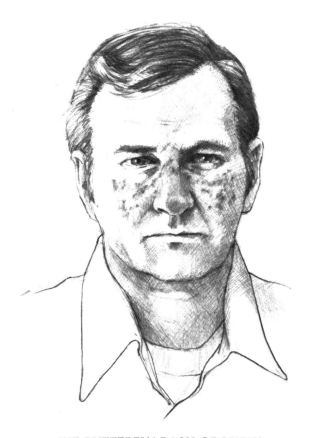

THE BUTTERFLY RASH OF LUPUS.

Once lupus has been diagnosed or strongly suspected, treatment may be started. Some patients may do superbly without any therapy at all. Others need drugs. At the outset, aspirin—as in other forms of arthritis—is the first to be tried. In mild cases, it may be enough to control the symptoms. Some physicians prefer to combine aspirin with other relatively innocuous antiarthritis agents. In more serious conditions, when aspirin is inadequate, experts will quickly turn to more potent drugs. The corticosteroid hormones like cortisone are used—and often used in large amounts. While these hormones are given in small doses for rheumatoid arthritis, they may be prescribed lavishly for lupus. The treatment must be individually fashioned for each patient and changed as the patient's condition requires.

The administration of these hormones in large amounts for periods of many months or years does not mean they are

55

given without caution. The adverse side effects of these substances are well known to physicians. They can cause swelling of the facial tissues in a form known as moon-face, bone softening, and mental changes, or they may activate a latent infection. Some of the hormone-induced mental changes may closely resemble those caused by lupus itself, and it is sometimes difficult to determine whether or not the drug is the actual offender.

As soon as possible, when the worst symptoms seem to be improving and blood tests show that the disease is being controlled, the daily dose of the hormone is reduced to the lowest effective level. In many instances, essentially all of the signs of the disease will disappear, and hormone treatment can be discontinued for months or years, and possibly forever. In most cases, the illness follows a mild, chronic course occasionally punctuated by a flare-up that usually can soon be controlled.

In patients who are sensitive to sunlight, hydroxy-chloroquine may be given for its value in protecting the skin from ultraviolet rays. The same drug may also be used for its anti-inflammatory action.

With the newly developed corticosteroids, and with our increasing knowledge of how to use them, many of the complications of lupus can be largely alleviated. Mental confusion will be cleared, chest pain is eased, rashes disappear, and even the hair grows back. Setting the proper dosage to maintain such improvement represents one of the most difficult problems for the physician. Yet it is a problem well worth solving because many of us have seen patients with a properly balanced program kept on daily doses of hormones safely and effectively for fifteen years or more.

Many corticosteroids are available. Some patients may be confused by the fact that one specialist will prescribe cortisone, another prednisone, and a third one of the newer and more expensive forms of corticosteroids. This is not to be taken as a sign that one prescription is proper and the others must therefore be wrong. It is recognized that all the hormones vary somewhat in safety and efficacy, and often in cost, but generally they yield the same clinical results. In the control of lupus, as in the therapy of many other diseases, physicians often prefer to use the product with which they are most familiar, and whose values and potential risks each knows best.

For those unusual patients who do not respond well even to hormones, there is still another class of drugs now being used experimentally. These are the immunosuppressive agents such as azathioprine, chlorambucil, and cyclophosphamide. They were introduced originally for the treatment of certain forms of cancer and have the ability to hold down unwanted immune reactions. Their use, too, is associated with serious risks, and they must be employed with exceptional caution.

It is probably impossible to say that any or all such treatments actually "cure" the disease. Even after a long period in which a patient has seemingly recovered from lupus, the condition can return, sometimes in serious form. This may happen when treatment is stopped too soon or when, without physician approval, the patient stops taking the prescribed drug.

Throughout, there must also be effective communication between patient and physician and between patient and family. There is almost always a need for reassurance, sympathy, support, and frank discussion. To combat the feelings of depression, fatigue, loneliness, anger, and fear, family members should attempt to provide support, but they should not be overly protective. On the other hand, they should not pretend that nothing has happened and that the patient is simply imagining all the problems. If ever arthritis is to be considered a disease that affects an entire family, this is unquestionably true of lupus. In addition, many people have found that they benefit greatly from meeting regularly with other lupus patients and sharing their problems, worries, and fears.

One record of the mounting success against this bizarre disease is the reduction in the reported death rates. Thirty years ago, less than 15 percent survived for as long as three years after diagnosis, and practically none lived for ten years. By 1954, the five-year survival rate had gone up to 50 percent; it rose to 70 percent in 1964, 80 percent in 1969, and 95 percent in 1976. In fact, in 1976, the reported ten-year survival rate was 92 percent. Even with severe kidney damage, once the most feared complication of lupus, the majority of victims survive. Such gratifying reports come not only from major medical centers, but from community hospitals as well.

Some of this improvement reflects better diagnostic

methods making it possible to detect more and milder cases. Some derives from better methods of treatment. Each year fewer deaths from lupus are being reported.

Thus, one of the most feared forms of disease can, in most cases, now be controlled. The important point to recognize is not only that more patients survive, but that, by taking reasonable precautions, they can hold virtually any kind of job, maintain a home, have children and raise a family, and follow an essentially normal life-style.

CHAPTER 7

CHRONIC ARTHRITIS IN CHILDREN

In the early 1900s, a distinguished British pediatrician described a form of arthritis that seemed to be as dreadful as it was rare. It produced clear signs of arthritic pain and inflammation in the joints of children. It also affected many other parts of the body. It could damage the eyes and even result in blindness. In a few cases, its complications were fatal. Fortunately, it appeared to be so uncommon that few physicians had ever seen a case. After the pediatrician who first reported it, Sir George Still, it was called Still's disease.

Now, under its modern name of juvenile rheumatoid arthritis—or, in some countries, chronic juvenile arthritis—it is known to be far more common and far less serious in the overwhelming proportion of cases. It is estimated to afflict 250,000 or more young patients in the United States. They become ill before the age of eighteen and some before the age of ten. With modern treatment that was not known in Still's time, it is almost never fatal, serious complications can be prevented in most instances, and the basic disease can usually be controlled. Sometimes the condition disappears, never to return.

Some highly skilled observers have recently reported that the disease occurs significantly more often among children of broken families—those in which there has been a separation, divorce, or death of a parent. It seems to happen more often in adopted children, and in children of unmarried mothers. On the other hand, many experts seem to have the impression that equally often it strikes children who come from what seem to be stable, strong, loving, emotionally balanced families.

In some patients, the disease begins with a salmon-colored skin rash that closely resembles that of measles. It

61

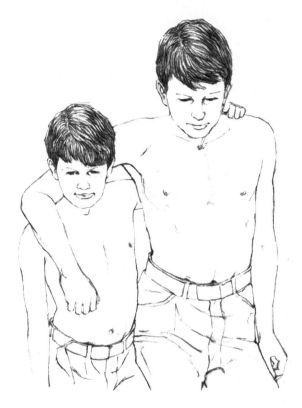

ARTHRITIS ATTACKS MORE CHILDREN EACH YEAR THAN DID
POLIO WHEN IT WAS MOST PREVALENT.

comes and goes in a matter of hours. Often it recurs daily
over a period of weeks. There is also a "spiking" fever; the
temperature may soar quickly to as high as 104 degrees and
then drop to normal, usually within a few hours. Both of
these signs may be present before inflammation, swelling,
and pain first appear in a joint.

Ordinarily, it is a benign form of arthritis, involving no
more than one or two joints. In some patients, however, the
disease progresses eventually to a form indistinguishable
from rheumatoid arthritis or ankylosing spondylitis. It is the
rare child who develops permanent involvement of the eyes,
spleen, lymph nodes, heart, and other organs. More than 90
percent of the patients do not have any such lasting
complications.

In reaching the proper diagnosis and deciding on the
appropriate course of treatment, the physician must exclude
a number of other diseases, including early ankylosing
spondylitis. X-ray examination and blood tests may help.

With or without treatment, most children will have a few remissions and then new flare-ups. Some of these flare-ups may appear long after the disease had apparently burned itself out.

Treatment for juvenile rheumatoid arthritis is usually the same as that for adult rheumatoid arthritis but even more conservative. It includes properly balanced rest and exercise, application of heat to alleviate pain and swelling, sometimes the temporary use of splints, and, uncommonly, surgery. As far as drug therapy is concerned, most experts are inclined to be even more cautious than they would be with adults. Aspirin or aspirinlike products are the basis of treatment. Some of the newer antiarthritis drugs have not been adequately tested in children; at least in the United States, the present drug regulation system makes it difficult or sometimes impossible to test any new drug adequately in children. Accordingly, investigators are unable to determine the correct dosage levels for young patients, the proper indications, and the important contraindications. Except in rapidly progressing cases, children are usually not treated with gold salts, hydroxychloroquine, or steroid hormones. Juvenile rheumatoid arthritis may itself limit bone growth; steroid hormones may have the same effect.

Many medical workers have stressed the need for diagnosis of the condition and start of treatment as quickly as possible. An important part of this early diagnosis involves a search for the beginning of any eye involvement. Usually such a study requires examination by a specialist. Unless eye treatment is begun promptly, there may be serious, lasting damage. With appropriate therapy, based on the administration of hormone eye drops, damage can almost always be prevented.

A quarter of a century ago, when many of today's physicians were completing their medical training, it was generally accepted that any child with what was then called juvenile rheumatoid arthritis should be packed off to bed and kept there for weeks or months. A similar routine was often utilized for adults with rheumatoid arthritis. It is now recognized that such treatment is needless and may be disastrous. First, most children ordered to stay in bed for prolonged periods will find ample reasons for getting out of bed; in technical terms, compliance with the doctor's orders is poor. Second, the unhappy psychological effects of enforced bed rest can far outweigh any physical benefits.

Today, most experts strongly recommend that children stay out of bed, go to school, and take part in recreational activities as much as possible.

A key part of the treatment is again a team effort that includes the physician and the two parents working closely together. Both the father and the mother must share the responsibility for seeing that the child follows the prescribed routine of rest, exercise, heat applications, and medication. Even more important, the father and the mother together must provide essential emotional support.

It is important to recognize that patients will have their good days or weeks and also their bad times. When things are not going well, the child may seem to be inexplicably tired, cross, angry, tearful, and completely uncooperative. At such times, the patient must have rest, exercise, heat, and medicine, and the parents must be patient and sympathetic.

On the other hand, the provision of patience and sympathy may go too far. Overprotecting or smothering a child with excessive concern at the wrong time can be destructive.

Such a problem is scarcely unique. It occurs in children with asthma and other chronic ailments. Occasionally, a family can benefit from professional psychological counseling and support, if only to get rid of unjustified guilt feelings and to cope with the feelings of jealousy or rejection exhibited by other children in the family.

The objective, as with normal children, is to help the patient grow up to become a normal, well-adapted adult to live in an adult world. With modern treatment, most young patients can achieve that goal.

CHAPTER 8

GOUT

*[Not Gluttony, Boozing,
or Wenching]*

In the seventeenth century, the English physician Thomas Sydenham penned this classical description of an acute attack of gout:

> The victim goes to bed and sleeps in good health. About two o'clock in the morning he is awakened by a severe pain in the great toe; more rarely in the heel, ankle or instep. This pain is like that of a dislocation, and yet the parts feel as if cold water were poured over them. Then follow chills and shivers, and a little fever. The pain, which was at first moderate, becomes more intense. With its intensity, the chills and shivers increase. After a time this comes to its height, accommodating itself to the bones and ligaments of the tarsus and metatarsus [in the foot]. Now it is a violent stretching and tearing of the ligaments—now it is a gnawing pain and now a pressure and tightening. So exquisite and lively meanwhile is the feeling of the part affected, that it cannot bear the weight of the bedclothes nor the jar of a person walking in the room.

As modern victims of gout can testify, Sydenham knew well whereof he wrote. The agony of even a single acute bout of gout can be remembered vividly after the passage of thirty years.

Accurately described since at least Greek and Roman times, gout reputedly attacks those with relatively high intelligence. Many victims have been famous historical figures: Achilles, Ulysses, Oedipus, Alexander the Great, Kublai Khan, Leonardo da Vinci, Michelangelo, the Medicis, Martin Luther, John Calvin, Henry VIII of England, Samuel Pepys, Samuel Johnson, Erasmus, John Milton, Isaac Newton, Charles Darwin, and Benjamin Franklin.

67

For many centuries, it was believed that gout is the punishment—well-deserved, of course—for over-indulgence in food, drink, or sex. Seventeenth- and eighteenth-century cartoonists typically portrayed the victim as the obese squire with his foot resting on a cushioned footstool and a bottle of port wine at his elbow. Sometimes a buxom serving wench was shown in the background.

The relationship between gout and port wine remains mysterious. The overindulgent patient might have gout and he also might drink port, but most observers apparently neglected to note that many gluttonous people did not suffer from gout, many gout victims were lean and abstemious, and many port drinkers had remarkably healthy big toes. Nonetheless, the gout-port connection has long been widely accepted. For instance, it is still stated that a 1703 treaty between England and Portugal lowering the import duty on port wines resulted in a vast increase in the incidence of gout among Englishmen. The supporting evidence is shaky. In our own work, we found some years ago in a survey of two hundred gout patients that nearly two-thirds had never used port or any other kind of wine before onset of their disease. Further, a preliminary study showed that, when victims of gout were given liberal amounts of port over long periods, they suffered no acute attacks.

Although the precise cause of gout is not known, the key chemical process is reasonably well understood. At the heart of the problem is apparently an inherited evolutionary mistake. Involved is a group of compounds known as purines, normally found in large amounts in such foodstuffs as sweetbreads, brains, kidneys, liver, heart, and even some grain products. In most lower species of animals, the purines are broken down by the body through a series of chemical steps culminating in the formation of *uric acid* and then *allantoin*. Allantoin is easily flushed out of the body through the kidneys and excreted as one component of urine. But in human beings and other higher forms—excluding, for some odd reason, the Dalmatian coachhound—the process stops at uric acid. And, in some people, uric acid is not so readily excreted. Its concentration builds up in the blood stream, and uric acid salt crystals are deposited in the joints, kidneys, and other areas. Deposits of these salts may appear in the outer rim of the ear and the elbow. In the past, large deposits of these uric acid compounds in the kidneys would often cause kidney damage and ultimately death.

In general, therefore, there is a close connection between high levels of uric acid in the blood and the deposit of urate salt crystals in the joints, where they can cause excruciating pain.

This seemingly direct cause-and-effect relationship, however, is not quite conclusive. Although most patients suffering from an acute attack of gout have high levels of uric acid in the blood, some people with similarly high uric acid levels have no gout problems at all. And some patients who never touch purine-rich foods—who avoid sweetbreads, kidneys, and the like—may have both high blood levels of uric acid and serious gout problems. It is now known that the body can form uric acid, even in excessive amounts, from a variety of nonpurine materials. This is not an altogether unusual situation; diabetic patients on a sugar-free diet can have abnormally high amounts of sugar in their blood, sugar formed from their own tissues or from noncarbohydrate foods.

Regardless of the source of uric acid, an excess can raise havoc in susceptible individuals, especially those with family histories of gout. In the United States, it is estimated that from half a million to a million individuals, and perhaps more (90–95 percent of them men) are afflicted. For the overwhelming majority, modern treatment has transformed their problem from a serious, disabling, crippling, painful, and sometimes life-threatening condition into a minor nuisance.

Although gout may strike first in one of the big toes, this happens in only about half the cases. It may begin in one of the other joints, such as the ankle or knee. Even without treatment, the attack may be over in a week or two. In many cases, there may not be another such experience for five or ten years or even longer. In most patients, however, there will be a second attack in perhaps six to twelve months, another a few months later, with shorter and shorter intervals between the events. There are instances in which the attack seems to have been set off by surgery, physical injury, excessive exercise, or the use of such drugs as diuretics and certain agents used to lower blood pressure. Alcoholic beverages in grossly excessive quantities may be responsible. But, for many patients, no triggering event is evident.

With modern treatment methods, it is unusual for patients to undergo frequent recurrences. If attacks do occur, they can usually be controlled within two days. Often attacks can be prevented. Two totally different therapeutic approaches are available, one for the acute attack and the other—termed interval treatment—to prevent or minimize future attacks.

To alleviate the pain of an attack, doctors since ancient times have utilized a plant product made from *Colchicum,* the autumn crocus, or its active ingredient, colchicine. Its use was introduced into the United States by that eminent gout victim Benjamin Franklin. This drug is so quickly effective and supposedly so specific that its action is sometimes thought to be diagnostic: if the patient is helped dramatically by colchicine, it has been claimed, the disease is almost always gout. More reliable confirmation is the finding of uric acid crystals in the inflamed joint.

In about 90 percent of patients, colchicine in adequate doses produces impressive relief of pain and swelling within six to twelve hours. In most cases, pain is completely gone within 48 hours.

Unfortunately, the effects of colchicine are not all good. Some 80 percent of patients also get significant cramps, diarrhea, nausea, or vomiting. As a result, many physicians have turned to indomethacin or phenylbutazone as the drug of choice in treating gout attacks. The new nonsteroid anti-inflammatory agents may also be effective. In this disease, aspirin and the corticosteroid hormones are seldom prescribed.

Obviously, exercise and laying on of hot compresses have no role in alleviating an acute attack. Either can make the unbearable pain even worse.

Aborting an acute attack is one thing. Preventing future bouts is something different. Three means must be considered for such "interval" therapy—a drug that will help the body excrete more uric acid through the kidneys; a drug that will limit the production of uric acid by the body; and diets low in purines. In addition, many patients may be protected by the daily use of colchicine in small doses.

Among the agents found valuable in helping to flush uric acid out through the kidneys (a group known technically as uricosuric drugs), the first to be developed and still one of the most widely used is probenecid, introduced in the 1960s. An even more recent uricosuric is sulfinpyrazone. Neither has any value in treating an acute attack, but both have a remarkable effect in removing abnormal stores of uric acid from the body, even deposits within a gouty joint. Neither is recommended for patients with histories of kidney stones or other kidney disease. A patient taking such drugs should be told to drink enough water so that he will excrete at least two quarts of urine each day.

Instead of using products like probenecid and sulfinpyrazone, or in instances in which they do not work or no longer work, physicians may turn to a drug that reduces the ability of the body to make uric acid. This approach results in lower levels of uric acid in the blood. The first such agent to appear on the market was allopurinol, introduced in the 1960s. It may be taken regularly for many years, possibly for life. Like the uricosuric drugs, it is useless in stopping an acute attack. It is indicated especially when uric acid stones have occurred in the kidneys.

None of these preventive drugs should be given until an acute attack is definitely over. Furthermore, some patients beginning such preventive treatment may undergo a temporary recurrence of an acute attack and may therefore need "protection" for a brief period with colchicine, phenylbutazone, or one of the other anti-inflammatory drugs.

The recommendation of an antigout diet is now infrequent. Few patients dine exclusively on such high-purine foods as sweetbreads, brain, and kidneys. As noted above, even if the patient eats no high-purine foods, uric acid is formed from normal body constituents. But there may be an occasional patient in whom the antigout drugs are inadequate, or who cannot tolerate them, and then a special diet may be considered.

The major question in preventive therapy is when to commence it. For a patient who probably will not suffer a second or third attack for many months or years, prevention seems needless—especially since an unexpected attack can be controlled with relative ease. At the other extreme, if the attacks seem to occur every few months or every few weeks, the institution of preventive maneuvers is more logical.

In the vast majority of cases, if patients carefully follow the prescribed routine, their gout will be a nuisance and sometimes an inconvenience, but no longer a catastrophe.

The routine, however, must be followed scrupulously. With few other chronic ailments is the future so much in the patient's own hands.

CHAPTER 9

INFECTIOUS ARTHRITIS

$\mathbf{B}$efore the introduction of the sulfa-drugs in the 1930s and penicillin in the early 1940s, infectious arthritis—the form caused by some invading microorganisms—represented a horror chapter in the arthritis story. Originating usually from a primary focus of infection, such as the sinus, lung, genital tract, or brain lining, bacteria would migrate through blood vessels and invade the knees, hips, ankles, or other joints. Precise diagnosis was sometimes difficult, and treatment frequently involved lengthy hospitalization and surgical intervention.

Today, with the availability of a wide assortment of antibiotics and other new antibacterial drugs, infectious arthritis is relatively easy to control and even to eradicate completely.

Ordinarily, the symptoms come on suddenly. Chills and fever are common, and the joint is painful and swollen. Sometimes diagnosis is easy. If the arthritis appears in a patient who is already known to be suffering from a streptococcus infection, gonorrhea, or meningococcal meningitis, for example, it is probable that the microbe responsible for the primary infection is also responsible for the infection in the joint. In some instances, however, the primary infection had not been even suspected and the identity of the causative organism was unknown. Often, the cause of the trouble can be determined by removing a sample of the synovial fluid from inside the joint space. The sample can be examined under a microscope, subjected to chemical tests, and incubated to determine which microbes are present.

Once the diagnosis is clear, it is usually possible to select the appropriate antibiotic. This is ordinarily given for the first few days by intravenous injection, in order to produce high concentrations in the blood, and later by oral administration. Most experts stress the need to commence treatment

75

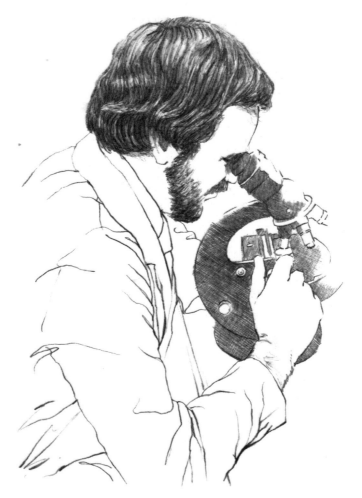

MICROSCOPIC EXAMINATION OF JOINT FLUID.

quickly. Treatment must be continued for at least 10 to 14 days and, in some cases, for a month. Delay or inadequate treatment can result in substantial and permanent joint damage, even within a period of a few days.

It must be stressed again that arthritic symptoms in a joint plus *moderate to high fever* call for action. One does not try aspirin for a week or two to see if the condition will go away by itself.

As with other forms of arthritis, the treatment usually includes bed rest, drug therapy to reduce pain, and sometimes the temporary application of splints. Surgical drainage may be needed. During convalescence, moderate exercise is commonly advised in order to preserve muscle tone and motion.

One thorny problem concerns infectious arthritis spreading from a primary gonorrheal infection. Until the advent of the sulfa drugs in the 1930s and then the antibiotics, gonorrhea and its various complications were all too common. Then gonorrhea decreased substantially, only to become common again with the introduction of oral contraceptives and changes in attitudes toward sexual behavior. Certainly during the past two decades, the resurgence of gonorrhea in adults has been a matter of grave concern. The problem has been notably serious among women. In men, the infection is usually detected quickly, since it is marked by an annoying but obvious discharge. In women, the discharge is by no means so apparent, and the infection may spread to one or more joints before it is diagnosed.

Recently, attention has been directed toward the involvement of viruses in infectious arthritis, notably the German measles virus. Arthritis can even occur after German measles vaccination. No antibiotic is useful against these forms, but usually they are self-limiting and do not cause any lasting damage.

Knowledgeable physicians will remain alert to the possible occurrence and the dangers of infectious arthritis, but they are aware that proper and prompt diagnosis and treatment will lead to virtually complete recovery in most patients.

CHAPTER 10

BURSITIS AND OTHER UNPLEASANTNESSES

The types of arthritis considered in the preceding chapters are probably the most common and potentially most serious forms of the disease. There are, however, others that are far from rare, each of which plagues tens or hundreds of thousands of victims. Some of them involve tissues outside of a joint.

Bursitis

A bursa is a closed saclike structure, usually filled with fluid, that cushions the movement of a muscle or tendon over a joint or other bony protuberance. Each is lined with a tissue closely resembling the synovial membrane lining a joint capsule.

If a bursa becomes seriously inflamed, the resulting bursitis and its tenderness and exquisite pain are something that the patient is not likely to forget. Rarely, it may require morphine injections for relief.

Bursitis frequently strikes in the shoulder, elbow, or hip. One type affects the bursa structures in the buttocks in those who are accustomed to sitting for prolonged periods and is known as "weaver's bottom." Another is commonly called "housemaid's knee." In many instances, there is no obvious explanation for the inflammation. In some patients, the bursitis appears to be triggered by a prolonged period of emotional tension. In others, it may be associated with rheumatoid arthritis or other inflammatory disease.

In some patients, recurring bursitis will almost invariably affect one area, such as the left shoulder or the right hip. In others, the condition seems to migrate, first hitting the right shoulder, for example, then a few months or a year later the left elbow, next the right hip, and so on.

If left untreated, the bursitis will generally subside in a few days or possibly one or two weeks. During that time, the pain can be excruciating, and motion of the affected parts becomes almost impossible. Only rarely does the inflammation continue indefinitely, leading to such a condition as "frozen shoulder."

Treatment often consists of immobilization, the application of warm or cold compresses, and the administration of such anti-inflammatory drugs as aspirin, indomethacin, and phenylbutazone. In some cases, physicians may inject a corticosteroid hormone directly into the inflamed bursa. This injection, by suppressing inflammation, may yield complete relief, sometimes within 24 hours, but the pain of the injection itself may be memorable. Experienced victims of bursitis (both authors of this book can be included in the category) will usually weigh carefully the pain of the illness against the possible pain of the injection before agreeing to that course of action.

Regardless of which treatment is used, exercise of the affected area—as soon as this is made possible by relief of pain—will usually enable the bursitis victim to resume normal motion.

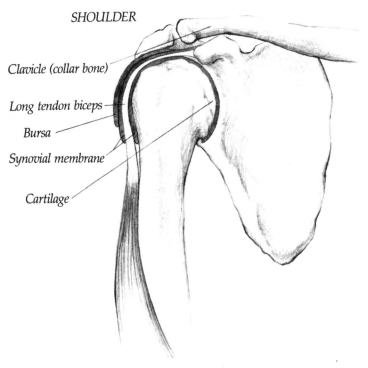

SHOULDER

Clavicle (collar bone)

Long tendon biceps

Bursa

Synovial membrane

Cartilage

LOCATION OF BURSA ADJACENT TO SHOULDER JOINT.

Sjögren's Syndrome

Most people are able to produce copious or at least adequate amounts of tears and saliva. Some are not, and are said to suffer from a condition often called "dry-eye." The eye surface becomes dry and irritated, and sometimes it is impossible for the victim to speak easily or to swallow. In a classical monograph published in 1933, the Swedish ophthalmologist Henrik Sjögren reported that dry-eye and its related difficulties are usually local manifestations of a systemic disease affecting the whole body.

Most of the victims are women, with a ratio of about nine women to one man. Among the systemic diseases that are associated with dry-eye are rheumatoid arthritis—perhaps one-third of all rheumatoid patients suffer from the eye and throat complications—and lupus.

Control is usually based on the frequent application of artificial tear drops to the eyes, perhaps every two or three hours, and the availability of water or other fluids to be sipped as needed.

Polymyalgia Rheumatica

Recognized as a form of rheumatic disease only about a decade ago, this puzzling and occasionally dangerous condition usually comes on abruptly in middle-aged or elderly patients, most of them women. Unlike rheumatoid arthritis or osteoarthritis, it almost never affects the hands or feet but strikes the shoulders and hips. There is prolonged and painful morning stiffness, and there may be fever and loss of weight.

Although there is a change in the blood sedimentation rate, which normally signals the presence of an inflammatory disease, it is not clear whether polymyalgia itself is a true form of inflammation.

The treatment is usually simple and the results are dramatic. It consists of the daily use of small amounts of corticosteroid hormones. If these do not work, the disease is probably not polymyalgia. In most cases, the condition seems to disappear after a year or two.

There is one complication that requires physicians to remain alert. In from roughly 5 to 10 percent of polymyalgia patients, inflammation may develop in the temporal arteries at each side of the forehead. If this condition is not detected quickly, often with the aid of a biopsy, and treated for about six months with large doses of steroid hormones, there may be sudden blindness. The cause of the blindness is an extension of the inflammation to the arteries that supply blood to the eyes.

Pseudogout

Mimicking true gout in most of its symptoms, false gout, or pseudogout, is marked by recurrent and exceedingly painful attacks in one or more joints. The big toe is rarely affected. It is most frequently the knee.

While gout is marked by the deposit of uric acid salt crystals in the joint, pseudogout results from the deposit of the calcium salt crystals of pyrophosphoric acid. It is uncommon in people under the age of sixty. Diagnosis usually depends on withdrawing a small amount of the joint fluid and detecting the microscopic crystals of the calcium salt.

Pseudogout is usually accompanied by the deposit of the calcium salts in the cartilage of the joint, and this condition—known as chondrocalcinosis—may be detected by x-ray studies.

For an acute attack of pseudogout, a physician will generally prescribe such anti-inflammatory agents as aspirin, indomethacin, phenylbutazone, or one of the corticosteroid hormones. Colchicine, long the standard remedy for gout, usually provides little benefit in pseudogout. The drugs used to prevent recurrent attacks of gout by lowering uric acid levels in the body have no value in the treatment of pseudogout.

Reiter's Syndrome

Another bizarre form of arthritis, Reiter's syndrome—named after the German bacteriologist Hans Reiter—can produce four different conditions:

An inflammation of the urethra, the tube carrying urine out of the bladder.

Conjunctivitis, or "pink eye."

Changes in the skin or mucous membranes, such as inflammation
    of the penis, pustulation of the skin resembling the patches
    characteristic of psoriasis, or inflammation of the mouth.

Arthritis, often in the knee or ankle.

Not all of these necessarily occur in the same patient at the same time.

Primarily a disease of young men, it may appear a few days or a few weeks after sexual intercourse. It may also appear, sometimes in epidemic form, after diarrhea caused by dysentery and other infections.

Such anti-inflammatory drugs as indomethacin and phenylbutazone are usually applied for relief of symptoms. The first attack is ordinarily self-limited, but recurrences are common.

It is believed that victims of Reiter's syndrome inherit a predisposition to the condition. Between approximately 80 and 90 percent of them carry the genetic marker HLA-B27 on their blood cells. This is the same marker that is found commonly in patients with "stiff spine," or ankylosing spondylitis. From 25 to 30 percent of Reiter's syndrome victims will ultimately develop "stiff spine."

Arthritis in Bowel Disease

Physicians have long been aware that some forms of intestinal inflammation may be accompanied by a painful but usually brief form of arthritis. Most common of these intestinal diseases are ulcerative colitis and inflammation of a part of the small intestine.

The arthritic complications may strike any joint in the body. When the bowel disease is in an acute stage, the arthritis is likely to be most severe. When the intestinal problem has been alleviated, the arthritis becomes less intense and usually disappears.

Treatment is generally the same as that for rheumatoid arthritis, although gold salts are never used. For most patients, drug therapy is required for only a few weeks or possibly months. Permanent deformity of arm or leg joints is rare.

In about 20 percent of the patients, however, the arthritis may later lead to "stiff spine." In such cases, the treatment will be that already described for ankylosing spondylitis. This spinal complication is probably predetermined by genetic factors.

Psoriatic Arthritis

As if psoriasis itself were not unpleasant enough, many psoriasis patients—perhaps one-quarter of them—are afflicted with arthritis, occasionally rheumatoid arthritis, but more commonly another type now classified as psoriatic arthritis.

In most cases, this form starts after the psoriasis has appeared. The two conditions, however, may start at the same time, or the arthritis may appear first. Usually the arthritis first attacks the end joints of the fingers, although it may strike other, larger joints.

Unlike other forms of arthritis, which may affect both hands, for example, or both feet, psoriatic arthritis is usually asymmetrical: that is, at least at the outset, it strikes only one hand or one foot.

Treatment of psoriatic arthritis is customarily the same as that for rheumatoid arthritis. If the spine becomes affected, the usual therapy for ankylosing spondylitis is applied. In addition, there is one drug that has a strategic place in psoriatic arthritis—an immunosuppressive agent known as methotrexate. Introduced first to control a relatively rare form of cancer, it was later applied—and applied enthusiastically—in the treatment of psoriasis. In many severe cases, it seemed to produce dramatic effects. In addition, possibly because of its immunosuppressive action, it seemed to control the arthritis of psoriasis. Although it is still being used, much of the enthusiasm for methotrexate has diminished. It may cause serious damage to the blood-forming organs, the liver, and other parts of the body, and its application calls for extreme caution.

This accounting by no means covers all the many forms of arthritis. Most of those not discussed here are relatively infrequent. In those uncommon forms, as with rheumatoid arthritis and osteoarthritis, the picture is not blissful. But it is certainly not hopeless. In nearly every instance, the disease can be controlled. Nearly every patient can be helped.

CHAPTER 11

THE DRUGS AGAINST ARTHRITIS

There is as yet no magic bullet for arthritis, a single drug that will completely and safely control, cure, or, ideally, prevent the disease. Possibly there never will be. The types of arthritis are so many, so complex, and so varied that it seems likely that a number of different causative processes are involved. The chances of finding a single chemical or vaccine effective in all cases appear to be exceedingly remote.

This is scarcely a unique situation. There is no one antibiotic or antibacterial agent that works against all infections. No single drug is good for all kinds of high blood pressure; nor is there a single chemical that has value against all the many forms of cancer.

In the case of arthritis, the modern advances in drug therapy have come from a number of developments:

The old hodge-podge of "arthritis" into which nearly all forms except gout were lumped at the start of this century has been divided and subdivided into scores of specific conditions by expert rheumatologists. In many instances, specific drugs— along with different types of rest, exercise, and the other parts of the treatment program—can be prescribed for the specific type of illness in which they can be most useful.

The modern physician has at hand an array of products, some of them introduced within the last twenty years and some within the last three, that have dramatically changed the complexion of drug treatment. Often they make possible a degree of arthritis control that was unachievable as recently as 1970.

Perhaps most important, physicians have developed new knowledge and new skills permitting them to use these drugs with maximum safety and maximum benefit.

89

In the use of all these products, old and new, there are certain key points that should be understood by physician and patient alike:

No arthritis drugs of any kind can be considered absolutely safe. Each has potential hazards. If used without appropriate safeguards, each can cause side effects ranging from annoying to fatal. Some of these adverse effects are rare or infrequent, while others—usually mild—are reported commonly. In the case of many stomach-irritating medications, the side effects can be minimized if the drug is taken with food or an antacid like magnesium or aluminum hydroxide. But not all such antacids deliver adequate relief, no matter what the advertising says.

With all drugs, it is essential for the patient to comply faithfully and precisely with the physician's instructions. Cutting down or stepping up the dosage, or skipping doses, without the knowledge and approval of the physician can have catastrophic consequences. In arthritis drug therapy, especially with the more powerful drugs, the patient who decides that, if three tablets a day are good, then nine a day must be three times as good, or who skips medication for two days and then triples the dosage on the third day, or who is told to use a drug for two weeks but keeps on taking it for four weeks "to give it a little more time to start working," or who "shares" it with a neighbor is inviting disaster. So is the patient with infectious arthritis who is told to take an antibiotic for four weeks but stops at the end of one because he or she "feels better."

Drugs alone can't do the whole job.

In general, depending upon the type of arthritis and the condition of the patient, the physician's choice of the proper drug will usually follow a pattern something like this:

Except for the treatment of gout and infectious arthritis, he will start with large doses of an aspirin-containing product, which may be all the patient will ever require. Many rheumatologists believe that, only when heavy dosages of aspirin do not give satisfying results after a trial of not much more than three months, stronger measures should be considered.

If aspirin is inadequate, or if the patient can't tolerate it, the physician will try one of the other nonhormonal drugs like fenopro-

90

fen, ibuprofen, hydroxychloroquine, indomethacin, naprox-
en, phenylbutazone, sulinac, or tolectin.*

In some cases of rheumatoid arthritis, it may be necessary to ad-
minister hydroxychloroquine, gold salts, or small doses of
corticosteroids.

In still more serious stages or forms of arthritis, certainly if the
disease appears to be uncontrolled, the physician may finally
turn to larger doses of one of the corticosteroid hormones or
penicillamine. In treating lupus, if aspirin is inadequate, the
physician may use corticosteroids at once.

In the special care of gout, the physician will base his prescribing
judgments on the nature, severity, and frequency of attacks.

Precautions should be taken with phenylbutazone, gold
salts, hydroxychloroquine, the corticosteroids, and penicillamine. Unless a physician is well-trained, experienced, and
competent to use these powerful but sometimes hazardous
compounds, consultation with an expert should be recommended to the patient—or the patient might well insist on it.

In large cities, such consultation is usually available
with relatively little difficulty. In smaller communities and
in rural areas, there may not be a rheumatologist or other
expert in the vicinity, and the consultation could involve the
burdensome inconveniences and expenses of travel. Such a
trip may be worthwhile; it could well minimize the risk of
needless pain, crippling, disability, and tissue damage, and
even needless death.

In the sections that follow, many of the most important
antiarthritis drugs now marketed in the United States will
be described, but no attempt has been made to cover all of
them. There are others—possibly scores—that are not approved in this country but can be obtained abroad. They are
not approved here for one simple reason: the Food and Drug
Administration, acting under the law, has ruled that not
enough substantial scientific evidence has been submitted
by the manufacturer to convince the FDA and its expert ad-
visors that the drug is both effective and relatively safe for
the intended uses. In the past, the FDA had been swayed by
testimonials from physicians: "It's a valuable drug," or "I
use it," or "I couldn't practice medicine without it." Since

* These are the generic names of the products. The brand names,
sometimes better known to patients, are given in the following sections.

the implementation of 1962 federal legislation, the FDA has no longer been impressed by endorsements; it now demands scientific proof. It may be noted, in this connection, that there is no impressive evidence that drugs approved in foreign countries but unapproved in the United States offer any substantial advantages. Although there is still controversy over the so-called drug lag, and the delays in obtaining FDA approval, most authorities advise against rushing overseas to get arthritis treatments that are not now available here.

A few drugs, notably the immunosuppressives and levamisole, are mentioned later in this chapter even though they have not been approved by the FDA for treating arthritis. They are, however, available on the market, having been approved for use in other diseases. With the knowledge and approval of the FDA, these agents are being tested experimentally on small groups of selected arthritis victims.

Finally there is a group of acetaminophen-containing products, most available without prescription, that are legally on the market and being used for arthritis treatment, though they are technically not antiarthritis drugs. They are recommended—often directly to the public—"for relief of the minor pains of arthritis." These acetaminophen products, such as Bromo Seltzer, Datril, Excedrin, Nyquil, Super-Anahist, Trigesic, Tylenol, and Vanquish, are unquestionably analgesic. They alleviate moderate pain, including the pain of arthritis. But pain is only one of the problems in arthritis. Acetaminophen products, unless they also contain an aspirinlike ingredient, have no demonstrated value in controlling inflammation or swelling. Arthritis can be a serious disease; it calls for carefully planned drug treatment.

Aspirin

Probably since prehistoric times, medicine men have known that fever can be relieved by administering an extract of willow bark or spiraea plants. The active substance, a salt of salicylic acid, was isolated a century and a half ago; its name comes from *Salix,* the botanical name for the willow. Its value in the control of fever was scientifically established in the 1870s, largely as a result of a blunder.

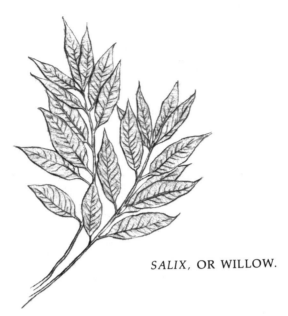

SALIX, OR WILLOW.

A decade earlier, Joseph Lister in England had revolutionized surgery by introducing a potent germ-killer called phenol, or carbolic acid. This powerful substance was of great value in preventing postsurgical infection, but it was far too toxic to be used internally for destroying microbes. In Germany, a distinguished chemist, Hermann Kolbe, therefore devised what he thought would be an ingenious way of getting around the problem. Working with a medical colleague, he proposed the administration of salicylic acid. His reasoning was simple: in the test tube, salicylic acid slowly breaks down to form phenol. The same thing, Kolbe reasoned, would happen in living tissue. It does nothing of the kind.

For a number of years, many physicians valiantly administered salicylic acid or its salts to victims of typhoid fever, typhus fever, pneumonia, and a variety of other infections. Regardless of Kolbe's idea, these patients proceeded to die in the usual numbers. For brief periods, however, they seemed to *feel* better.

In 1875, working in a Swiss hospital, Carl Emil Buss provided the explanation: regardless of what it did or did not do to invading microbes, salicylic acid almost always reduced fever. It was the first effective fever-fighter to be introduced since quinine-containing cinchona bark was brought from Peru to Europe in the seventeenth century.

A year after Buss reported his findings, the second major step was taken when a German army doctor, Franz Stricker, announced the discovery that the salicylates could do more than reduce fever. At least temporarily, they could alleviate some of the symptoms of arthritis.

Regrettably, although these substances were undeniably effective against fever and—in large amounts—against arthritis, they were all too often intensely irritating to the stomach. This problem was largely solved by another German scientist, Felix Hoffmann of the Bayer Company, who discovered (or actually rediscovered) a derivative called acetyl salicylic acid. Among the first patients to benefit from the new product was Hoffmann's own father, who had been an arthritis victim for years—and who had bitterly complained all those years about the way that ordinary salicylates ruined his stomach. Acetyl salicylic acid was introduced to medicine in 1899 under the name of aspirin, a name taken from *a-* (for acetyl) and *spirin* (from the name of the spiraea plant). Its formal introduction was made by Heinrich Dreser, head of Bayer's drug research laboratory.

Dreser is well known to drug experts for another reason. It was he who also introduced acetyl morphine for the treatment and perhaps cure of morphine addiction. Its value against morphine addiction was said to be so heroic that Dreser named it heroin.

In recent years, the obvious toxic side effects of aspirin have been widely publicized, and many people have been warned of the fact that aspirin and related products can cause nausea, vomiting, sometimes intense stomach irrita-

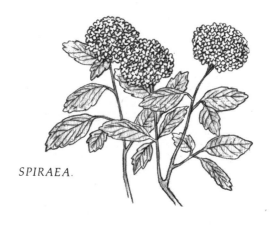

SPIRAEA.

tion and pain, ulceration, even bleeding. It may also induce hearing loss. Although these undesirable effects may occur with the use of small doses, they are more likely to happen with the ingestion of the large doses often required in arthritis treatment to control inflammation. In exceedingly large doses, aspirin can cause death. Fatal aspirin poisoning in small children who gain access to home medicine cabinets has been distressingly common. For this reason, aspirin is often bottled now in containers with "childproof" caps. Patients with hands so badly affected by arthritis that they cannot cope with such safety devices can have the pharmacist substitute a standard container.

As any pharmacy or supermarket shopper is aware, aspirin is currently marketed in many forms and under a multitude of names. By and large, the products are essentially the same, although their prices may vary considerably. Most of these products contain aspirin in 5-grain tablets.

One exception is so-called buffered aspirin, in which the active ingredient is combined with an antacid substance to minimize stomach irritation. Patients can usually prevent such irritation at less expense by taking the drug with food or with an inexpensive antacid. Doses so large that they cause ringing in the ears should be avoided. Those who already have poor hearing or whose hearing ability is decreasing may be at particular risk, because they may be unable to hear any ringing sounds; unquestionably, they should limit their aspirin intake.

Another exception is Anacin, which contains $6\frac{2}{3}$ rather than 5 grains of aspirin and includes caffeine as well. There seems to be no scientific evidence that caffeine has any effect in the treatment of arthritis. With its higher content of aspirin, such a product may be taken in fewer doses each day. Its retail cost as based on equivalent quantities of aspirin, however, is substantially higher than that of ordinary 5-grain tablets. Other extrastrength products are available, but may not be worth the added cost.

Some widely advertised preparations are said to get into the blood stream more rapidly and thus offer quicker relief. Such a characteristic may have value for the rapid relief of headache, but it has no significance in the day-long control of inflammation.

Other widely promoted products combine aspirin with such antipain remedies as acetaminophen and salicylamide.

95

There appears to be no scientific proof that any of these has a greater antiarthritis action than the same amount of aspirin taken alone. Most physicians have shown little enthusiasm for various aspirin products that are coated with substances intended to reduce stomach irritation in arthritis treatment. Some of these products may possess certain advantages, but in others the coating may interfere with the absorption of aspirin from the digestive tract.

The relative cost of aspirin and other antiarthritis products as based on average expenditure per month is shown in the table beginning on page 122.

During the last part of the nineteenth century and the first of the twentieth, many other synthetic substances, some of them related to aspirin, were widely prescribed for arthritis. Among them were antipyrine, acetanilide or antifebrin, phenacetin, and pyramidon or aminopyrine. Phenacetin is still used in a number of remedies, mainly for the control of fever and headache. Primarily because of their hazards or their limited effectiveness, however, the others are either no longer used or limited to minor applications. In the United States, phenacetin is a component of numerous combination products, many of which can be described as shotgun remedies.

Phenylbutazone

One of the aspirin-related compounds found early to be highly effective in the treatment of fever, pain, and some forms of arthritis was the substance named pyramidon or aminopyrine. Widely marketed at one time, it later fell into disfavor as its serious toxic effects became apparent.

Before its popularity declined, it was administered only in the form of tablets to be taken by mouth. Some physicians in Europe felt a need for the drug to be put into solution so that it could be given by intramuscular injection. Unfortunately, aminopyrine is not easily soluble. To overcome this problem, it was mixed with another close chemical relative called phenylbutazone, which had been synthesized in 1946 by chemists in the Geigy Laboratories in Basel, Switzerland. The injectable combination worked well—in fact, better than aminopyrine alone—and was quickly marketed in Europe under the name of Irgapyrin and in the United States as Butapyrin.

Only after the introduction of the combination was it discovered that its greater value was due to the added ingredient, phenylbutazone, and the other ingredient, aminopyrine, was not important. Since 1952, phenylbutazone* has been available for general use and has been accepted particularly for the treatment of such forms of arthritis as acute gout and ankylosing spondylitis.

Although phenylbutazone is more effective than aspirin for these conditions, it carries well-demonstrated risks, especially gastric irritation, and serious and even irreversible damage to the blood-forming organs. In order to minimize gastric irritation, many physicians prescribe phenylbutazone in combination with antacids or recommend that it be taken with food. Fortunately, the effects on the blood are rare. Physicians will usually order blood tests if treatment must continue for more than a week or two. Experts warn, however, that not even periodic blood tests will make it possible to prevent serious damage in all cases.

Indomethacin

In the early 1960s, a group of Merck scientists was seeking to find an antiarthritis agent more effective than aspirin and some of the other early drugs but less hazardous than the corticosteroid hormones. For their study, they selected a series of synthetic compounds containing the so-called indole nucleus. There were two reasons for choosing the indole derivatives. First, there were suggestions that some arthritis patients had an abnormal way of metabolizing tryptophane—an indole-containing amino acid in proteins. (It later became apparent that this had nothing to do with arthritis.) Second, they had a number of indole derivatives left over from an earlier investigation that also had nothing to do with arthritis.

The Merck group, headed by chemist Tsung-Ying Shen and pharmacologist Charles Winter, developed a screening technique that consisted of implanting an inflammation-causing material under the skin of a rat and then studying the effect of the test drug.

* Marketed by Ciba-Geigy under the brand name of Butazolidin and by other companies as phenylbutazone. A related substance is marketed by Ciba-Geigy under the brand name of Tandearil and by other companies as oxyphenbutazone.

Eventually the scientists synthesized and tested more than 14,000 compounds. One of the first to be developed—and the third to be tried on patients—was indomethacin. It was synthesized in 1963, given to the first patient, an Ohio school teacher, in that same year, and put on the market in 1965.*

One of the early users of the drug was another Merck investigator who himself had osteoarthritis of the hip. "He was in such bad shape," recalls Dr. Winter, "that he couldn't walk from the parking lot into the building. So he got a special permit from the company to allow his wife to drive right up to the door of the building. When indomethacin was in the trial stage, I told him about it. Well, about two days later I was coming to work in the morning and here he was, walking from the parking lot into the building."

Most experts would agree that indomethacin relieves pain and reduces fever, swelling, and tenderness of an inflamed joint. It is generally more effective than aspirin. A common side effect is headache, which calls for a lower dose or the selection of a different drug. It can also produce from moderate to severe gastrointestinal effects, although these may be minimized by taking the drug with food or antacids.

Indomethacin has been found to be particularly effective in treating patients who have ankylosing spondylitis or severe osteoarthritis of the hip, or who are suffering an acute attack of gout.

The Newer Nonsteroidal Anti-Inflammatory Agents

Within the space of about four years, five new anti-inflammatory drugs won FDA approval for marketing—ibuprofen in 1974, fenoprofen, naproxen, and tolmetin in 1976, and sulindac in 1978. They have no chemical relationship to cortisone and the other steroid hormones.

Two of them, naproxen and tolmetin, were approved for use only against rheumatoid arthritis. Ibuprofen, feno-

---

* Marketed under the brand name of Indocin by Merck Sharp & Dohme.

profen, and sulindac were approved for the treatment of
rheumatoid arthritis and osteoarthritis. In addition, the FDA
approved sulindac for use in "acute painful shoulder," ankylosing spondilitis, and acute gout.

All of them are, without doubt, useful in the control of
arthritic inflammation. All are effective, at least in some patients, but probably no more so than aspirin and certainly
more expensive. All can have disagreeable side effects. They
may, however, be useful for those who cannot tolerate
aspirin.

Currently, the advantages of these products over aspirin
are a matter of some dispute, as are the relative advantages
and disadvantages among the five drugs themselves. A few
enthusiasts have suggested that they are so much better than
aspirin that the latter should no longer be considered the
standard drug of first choice. Most experts, however, feel
that no such decision can yet be made. It seems that not all
patients respond in the same way to each of the new products. It is also probable that none of these substances has
been used long enough to allow final evaluation.

Ibuprofen. The first of these new nonsteroidal anti-
inflammatory substances to appear was ibuprofen.* Its discovery culminated a fifteen-year research program by a
British firm, the Boots Pure Drug Company of Nottingham.
Used in the United Kingdom since 1969, it is marketed in
the United States under a license from Boots to the Upjohn
Company, which itself spent twelve years on research.

Fenoprofen. For many years, scientists at the Lilly laboratories had demonstrated a keen interest in developing improved drugs for the control of pain. From this research came
propoxyphene (Darvon), which has been widely prescribed
for many painful conditions. Propoxyphene, however, has
no value in the treatment of inflammation and similar aspects of arthritis.

Looking for a chemical that would be effective against
inflammation, the Lilly workers used an ingenious new
test-tube method to screen many thousands of substances
and came up with only a few that seemed worthy of testing

* Marketed in the United States under the brand name of Motrin by
Upjohn.

in experimental animals. One of these, known as the "lead" compound, was particularly intriguing; oddly enough, it had been involved in earlier studies aimed at the control of blood cholesterol levels, but its anti-inflammatory actions had been unsuspected.

From this lead compound, nearly 300 derivatives were synthesized and subjected to additional testing in animals. The best of these new substances was fenoprofen,* with the greatest degree of activity and the fewest side effects. Approval for testing fenoprofen in human beings was given by the FDA in 1969, and the drug was cleared for marketing seven years later.

Naproxen. Discovery of naproxen† was first announced by the Syntex laboratories in 1970. By that time, human testing was already underway, first mainly in Mexico City and later elsewhere in Latin America, Europe, and the United States. The clinical tests confirmed the results of laboratory studies indicating that the drug would be effective in the control of pain, fever, and inflammation. In rheumatoid arthritis patients, it alleviates joint pain, joint swelling, and morning stiffness.

The drug is so long-acting that most patients need to take it only twice daily.

First marketed in Mexico in 1972, naproxen was approved for use in the United States in 1976.

Tolmetin. One of about 200 different compounds specifically designed by McNeil to combat inflammation and pain, tolmetin‡ was synthesized in 1967 and, after two years of animal experimentation, was found to be the most useful of the new chemicals. Human testing began in 1969, and FDA approval was granted seven years later.

Sulindac. Developed under the direction of the same Merck scientists who created earlier antiarthritis drugs, sulindac§ is

---

* Marketed under the brand name of Nalfon by Dicta, a division of Eli Lilly.

† Marketed under the brand name of Naprosyn by Syntex.

‡ Marketed under the brand name of Tolectin by McNeil Laboratories.

§ Marketed under the brand name of Clinoril by Merck Sharp & Dohme.

a member of a group of chemicals called indenes. It is related to indomethacin. Like naproxen, it is long-acting and needs to be taken only two times a day. The most common side effect is gastrointestinal distress.

Hydroxychloroquine

During World War II, a major research program was set up in the United States to develop synthetic substitutes for quinine needed for the treatment of malaria. In this study, which continued long after the end of hostilities, a number of new compounds were synthesized, screened on experimental animals, and then released for field trials on human subjects. One of the best of these was chloroquine, or Aralen, a remote relative of quinine. (It was learned later that the same drug had already been discovered by German scientists.) To measure its safety, it was tested on a group of prison volunteers by University of Chicago investigators. It turned out to be quite safe. Also, it was noted, some of the prisoners had been suffering from arthritis, and the chloroquine helped their arthritis symptoms. At about the same time, British physicians used the drug on malaria patients—some of whom also happened to have arthritis—and demonstrated that the arthritis symptoms were alleviated.

From 1957 to 1971, chloroquine was approved for use in the treatment of arthritis. A superior derivative, hydroxychloroquine,* has been in use since 1958. The latter is used in treating mild to moderate cases of rheumatoid arthritis and mild to moderate lupus when safer agents are inadequate. It can produce adverse side effects, however, especially eye damage. Thus, for patients taking hydroxychloroquine, periodic eye examinations are essential. The drug is also used to protect the skin of sun-sensitive lupus patients from ultraviolet rays.

Gold Salts

For two thousand years or more, gold and gold compounds have had questionable acceptance as useful drugs. Convinc-

* Marketed under the brand name of Plaquenil by Winthrop.

ing evidence of their value, however, was hard to find. Then, in the last half of the nineteenth century, gold salts—along with salts of other heavy metals like mercury, lead, silver, and antimony—were subjected to more careful examination.

Some investigators, most of them in Germany, reported that gold salts were clearly valuable in combating tuberculosis and other infections.

The next steps were presumably logical: gold controlled infections, rheumatoid arthritis was probably caused by an infection, and therefore gold should control arthritis, which it did in some cases. It was all very reasonable, except that later and more careful studies have failed—at least, so far—to demonstrate any infectious cause for rheumatoid arthritis.

Described by German workers during the late 1800s and early 1900s, the gold treatment for arthritis was established on a more scientific basis by a French investigator, Jacques Forestier, in 1929. Although its early use was controversial, probably because of the administration of excessively high dosages with resultant toxicity, the gold treatment is now frequently applied in both adult and juvenile rheumatoid arthritis, especially when the disease is flaring and safer drugs are inadequate.

Two major gold products are generally used, aurothioglucose and gold sodium thiomalate.* Both are given by weekly intramuscular injections in a course of treatment that usually lasts for many months. British reports suggest that the patient's condition may become worse about a year after the treatment is complete. Relapse is less likely if gold injections are continued indefinitely at increasingly greater intervals. The results are far from dramatic, and it may take three or four months for them to be apparent, but they do appear in most patients, especially if the onset of the disease was only a few years earlier. Adverse reactions, notably skin rash and a sore mouth and sometimes involving the blood-forming organs and the kidneys, have been reported to occur in about 30 percent of the patients. Thus, the physicians of many patients will seek another opinion before embarking on the treatment. It is essential that there be weekly or biweekly blood counts and urine tests to detect early signs of toxicity.

* Aurothioglucose is marketed under the brand name of Solganol by Schering, and gold sodium thiomalate under the brand name of Myochrysine by Merck Sharp & Dohme.

Treatment with gold is expensive. A course of about twenty injections, together with office visits, tests and analyses, and the preliminary consultation, is estimated to cost $600.

Penicillamine

In 1977, a national publication splashed coast-to-coast a gaudy account of the "fantastic" results of penicillamine in the treatment of arthritis.

Perhaps the person most distressed by the report was Dr. Israeli Jaffe of New York Medical College, who for fifteen years had been conducting cautious, painstaking research on the value of the drug in treating rheumatoid arthritis. "Making it sound almost as easy to get as chewing gum," he said at a press conference, "was a cruel disservice to arthritis sufferers."

A derivative of penicillin, penicillamine* has no value as an antibiotic but has been approved in many countries—including the United States—for the treatment of Wilson's disease, a rare affliction due to excess retention of copper in the body.

Studies by Jaffe and other investigators have shown that penicillamine is effective in relieving the inflammation and pain of rheumatoid arthritis. It has been proposed for administration to patients for whom gold treatments and small doses of a corticosteroid hormone do not work, or to patients who cannot tolerate them. Like the gold salts, it is slow to take effect, and it may require twelve weeks or longer to determine if it will have any value.

Unfortunately, as Jaffe and others have found, the undoubted benefits of penicillamine are counterbalanced by an assortment of potential side-effects, some so serious as to require persistent vigilance to avoid a serious drop in blood components and other dangerous and even lethal reactions.

An official of the Arthritis Foundation, who herself was given penicillamine as an experimental drug, put it this way: "Like the girl with the curl, when penicillamine is good, it's very, very good, but when it's bad . . . well, watch out."

* Marketed by Merck Sharp & Dohme under the brand name of Cuprimine and scheduled for marketing in 1979 by Wallace Laboratories under the brand name of Depen.

Used in other countries since 1973 for the treatment of arthritis, it was approved by the FDA in late 1978 for administration to rheumatoid arthritis patients.

The Corticosteroids

Among the most fascinating hormone-secreting glands in the body are the adrenals, two small organs perched above the kidneys. The inner part of each gland is the source of epinephrine, or adrenalin. The outer shell, or cortex, is the source of the family of adrenal corticosteroid hormones. The discovery, separation, synthesis, and introduction of these corticosteroids mark one of the major breakthroughs in twentieth-century medicine.

During the 1930s, crude extracts of the corticosteroids made from animal glands were used in the treatment of adrenal insufficiency, also known as Addison's disease, enabling many patients to get temporary relief from the life-threatening illness. Basic research on the substances was undertaken by a few scientists in research centers and pharmaceutical companies, but the field was considered of little practical importance.

What suddenly changed this situation was a rumor that circulated in Washington, D.C., in the fall of 1940 and the early months of 1941. An extract of adrenal corticosteroids, it was said, was enabling pilots in the Nazi *Luftwaffe* to fly and engage in combat at altitudes of as much as 40,000 feet, and German submarines were busily plying the Atlantic bringing adrenal glands from Argentine slaughterhouses for preparation of the extracts. The rumors later turned out to be untrue, but they were enough to stimulate action among the researchers.

The investigations of the 1930s had indicated that the batch of corticosteroids in adrenal cortex extract included at least six individual substances, named Compounds A, B, C, D, E, and F, in the sequence in which they had been isolated. All are complicated in molecular structure and difficult to obtain in adequate amounts from animal glands. At the outset, they were difficult if not impossible to synthesize in the laboratory. Compound E, which was eventually to receive the most attention, had been isolated and its structural formula worked out independently and almost simultaneously by Edward Kendall at the Mayo Foundation laboratories and Tadeusz Reichstein of the University of Basel in Switzerland. Much later, historians were intrigued to find these words written in a Mayo laboratory notebook: "Try Compound E in rheumatoid arthritis." The entry was dated April 1941 and written by Dr. Philip Hench, then the top rheumatologist at the Mayo Clinic.

Hench's inspired hunch came from repeated conversations with Kendall about the fact that many women suffering from rheumatoid arthritis show striking improvement during pregnancy. The pain clears, stiffness is lessened or disappears, and the inflammation is significantly reduced, only to reappear at the end of the pregnancy. And, during pregnancy, there are changes in hormone production by the adrenals. Seven years passed, however, before the Mayo physician could test his idea; in 1941, there was not enough Compound E available to cover the head of the proverbial pin.

The first of the corticosteroids to be produced in any significant amount was Compound A. Using the starting chemicals available to them, scientists at the Merck Laboratories synthesized a small supply of Compound A for testing in animals. It turned out to be a dud. The Merck group, headed by Lewis Sarett and working closely with Kendall, next synthesized small amounts of Compounds E and F. Compound E was effective against Addison's disease, but Compound F was better.

The scientists had synthesized only nine grams of Compound E, less than one-third of an ounce. Six grams were assigned to physicians for studies on Addison's disease. The rest was doled out in very small quantities for chemical investigation. Then Hench asked for a supply, and a small amount was sent to him at the Mayo Clinic. Compound E was soon to win worldwide acclaim under the name of cortisone. Without that "small amount" made available for the Mayo study, the value of cortisone in arthritis might have remained undiscovered for years and perhaps decades.

On the evening of September 21, 1948, the first injection of 50 milligrams—half of the proposed 100-milligram daily dose—was given to a twenty-nine-year-old woman who had been suffering from rheumatoid arthritis and was virtually bedridden. It was only with great difficulty that she was able to turn over in bed without assistance.

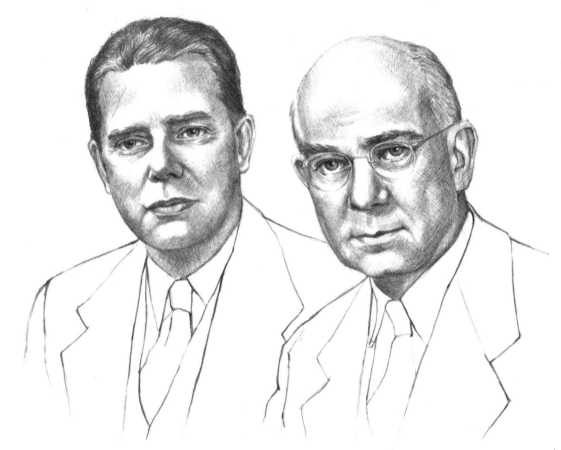

PHILIP HENCH AND EDWARD KENDALL, PIONEERS IN CORTISONE RESEARCH.

The report of her case by Hench and his associates, Drs. Charles Slocumb and Howard Polley, along with Kendall, is memorable:

She was admitted to the Clinic and the hospital on July 26, 1948. Many joints were stiff, swollen, tender, and painful on motion. Roentgenograms [x-ray photographs] revealed destructive changes in her right hip, because of which she limped, and less extensive changes in other joints. . . .
On September 20 the patient's joints were worse than they had been. On September 21 she could hardly get out of bed. On that day we began the daily intragluteal [in the buttock] injection of 100 mg. of Compound E. During that day no change was apparent;

walking was so painful that she ventured only once
from the room. . . . But when she awoke on September
23, she rolled over in bed with ease, and noted much
less muscular soreness. On September 24, painful
morning stiffness was entirely gone. Scarcely able to
walk three days previously, the patient now walked
with only a slight limp. . . .

By September 27, a week after the administration of
Compound E was begun, articular as well as muscular
stiffness had almost completely disappeared, and
tenderness and pain on motion, and even swellings,
were markedly lessened. The next day she shopped
downtown for three hours, feeling tired thereafter, but
not sore or stiff. . . .

Hench telephoned his friends at Merck. "Get us more cortisone," he said.

On the strength of the results for this first patient, and of
those for a second and a third, whose improvement was
similarly dramatic, Merck decided to go ahead with production on the basis of what was described afterwards as involving "the most expense, the sheerest faith, and the least evidence in the history of drug manufacturing." For the job, the
company assembled the largest task force in its history.

There were two particular problems. Although the won-
ders of cortisone made headlines throughout the world, with
accounts of patients dancing in the wards, the hormone offered no cure for arthritis, and its use could result in serious
side effects. Howard Polley, one of the original Mayo team,
said later:

The press and the public simply ran away with the
story. We knew within less than two months that
cortisone had severe side effects in the dosage used
initially. Moreover, cortisone was never proposed by us
as a cure, in the sense that antibiotics can eradicate an
infection. . . . Unfortunately, as a result of earlier
unrestrained enthusiasm, the cart got put before the
horse.

Regardless of the limitations, the discovery of the remarkable anti-inflammatory effects of cortisone and two
other hormones was enough to win a Nobel Prize for Hench,
Kendall, and Reichstein in 1950.

107

The second problem concerned the practical matter of production and costs. The need for cortisone was so great that it could not be filled even if all the adrenal glands from all the slaughterhouses in the world could be collected. The only solution was to develop a synthetic process—or, more realistically, a series of synthetic processes—using readily available starting materials. The original Merck procedure, beginning with a chemical from cattle bile, consisted of thirty-seven separate steps. It was described as extremely complicated, with a pathetically small yield, and horrendously expensive. In the first year or two, Merck managed to produce 400 grams of cortisone—enough to treat sixty-six patients for what was then only a two-month treatment period, at a cost of $200 per gram, or more than $1,200 per patient. By late 1952, the Merck chemists improved the procedure to the point at which the cost of cortisone was down to $35 per gram, but it seemed all too obvious that the process was still not suitable for mass production.

A major difficulty was to find a suitable starting material in adequate amounts at a reasonable price. Merck's original procedure beginning with cattle bile could not fill the bill. Various scientists considered beginning with raw materials from soy beans or yeast. Some investigators read with interest about the seeds of a particular species of African vine known as *Strophanthus* and described in the nineteenth century by Dr. David Livingstone (of "Dr. Livingstone, I presume" fame). At least six expeditions were dispatched to Africa, but none could locate the proper species. An ideal starting material would be a well-known sex hormone, progesterone, but progesterone—if any could be found—was priced at about $35,000 a pound wholesale.

After a few years of intensive work, two major improvements were recorded. Scientists at the Upjohn Laboratories discovered that the original thirty-seven-step Merck procedure could be drastically shortened by taking advantage of a simple mold fermentation, which could replace complicated chemical maneuvers. And, in Mexico City, investigators at the then almost-unheard-of pharmaceutical company called Syntex announced that they could start with a compound extracted from a wild yam root and turn it into progesterone, delivering at least a ton per month at a price of about $200 a pound. At about the same time, Merck further improved its procedure for synthesizing cortisone and other

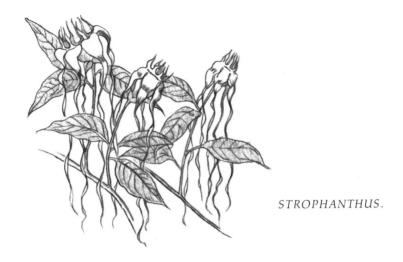

STROPHANTHUS.

steroid hormones, and other firms developed their own processes. The production bottleneck had been cleared. Corticosteroid treatment now costs as little as from five to twenty-five cents per patient per day, depending on the dosage and the particular hormone prescribed.

In the past quarter-century, the corticosteroids, employed in the treatment of arthritis and many other diseases, have grown from a few naturally occurring substances to a dozen or more products, most of them creations of modern chemistry. Among them are cortisone itself, hydrocortisone (originally called Compound F), and synthetic prednisone.* Numerous other synthetic products, most of them still under patent and somewhat more expensive, are also used.

The relative advantages and disadvantages of all these products are currently a matter of some controversy, at least among the manufacturers who market them. Some physicians believe that the new synthetic hormones are worth their extra cost because they are somewhat more effective and less hazardous under certain circumstances. Other physicians are not convinced. It is probable that the inherent benefits and hazards of the drugs are less important than the skill and judgment of the physicians who prescribe them. It

* Hydrocortisone is marketed under many brand names by many firms and under its generic name by a number of generic drug companies. Prednisone was marketed first under the brand name of Meticorten by Schering; now it is marketed under several brand names and its generic name by various firms.

is they who decide when it is time to use them, what the lowest effective dosages are that can be safely employed, and for how long.

Originally, cortisone and hydrocortisone were given only by injection. Our group at the University of California, San Francisco, was among the earliest to find that these hormones could be put in solution, properly flavored (with raspberry, strawberry or cherry) and taken orally.

For patients in whom certain of these compounds can be effective when given by direct injection into a joint, perhaps a few times a year, the corticosteroids can produce dramatic results. Side effects do not generally occur. For patients to whom the drugs are administered orally—the most commonly employed method—they can also be dramatically effective but not without adverse effects if used injudiciously. Among the potential side effects related to dosage and duration of treatment are moon-face, bone softening, growth of excessive facial hair, high blood pressure, eye problems, lessened resistance to tuberculosis and other infections, either bacterial or viral, the masking of infection, and psychotic changes.

ACTH

Shortly after recognition of the anti-inflammatory action of cortisone, a totally different but nonetheless related substance was found to have the same effect in patients with rheumatoid arthritis and other conditions. Known as adrenocorticotropic hormone, or ACTH, it is secreted by the pea-sized pituitary, referred to as the master gland, located on the underside of the brain, just above the roof of the mouth. The pituitary produces a number of different hormones, each of which regulates the hormone production of another gland—that is, production of the female sex hormones by the ovaries, the male sex hormones by the testes, insulin by the pancreas, thyroid hormone by the thyroid, and the corticosteroids by the adrenal cortex. As a treatment for arthritis, injection of ACTH causes the adrenal glands to increase their secretion of natural corticosteroids, which in turn may relieve the symptoms of the disease.

As a result of impressive research at university centers, particularly a project headed by Choh Hao Li at the University of California, and at the Armour Laboratories, practical techniques were developed for isolating ACTH from hog and beef pituitaries. Few physicians today favor the use of ACTH in treating arthritis. Most do not feel that ACTH has any important advantages, and it has the disadvantages of having to be given by injection and possibly causing a reaction to a "foreign protein." Like the corticosteroids, ACTH usually yields only temporary relief.

Despite the complexities of treating arthritis with corticosteroids or ACTH, their judicious use may mean the difference between a patient who is self-supporting and one who is totally dependent on others, and sometimes the difference between life and death.

It is difficult to realize that until recently physicians attempted to cope with certain forms of arthritis without these hormones. It is even more difficult to realize how they managed.

Experimental Drugs

Under the watchful observation and control of the FDA, a number of quite different drugs are now being tested for their effectiveness against arthritis. In some foreign countries, several of these drugs have received governmental approval for use in treating various conditions, including arthritis. In the United States, some are already on the market, but the treatment of arthritis is so far not approved by the FDA. In fact, one of these products has been approved only for veterinary use.

By the end of 1978, it was impossible to predict when or if any of these drugs will be added to the list of approved arthritis remedies.

The Immunosuppressives.   Mustard gas, applied with devastating effects during World War I, was described as one of the most hideous chemical warfare agents used in the battles in Europe. Developed for World War II, but apparently never used in combat, a derivative known as nitrogen mustard was probably more deadly. As a result of a freakish accident, some British troops on a torpedoed ship were exposed to nitrogen mustard that had spilled into sea water.

111

The exposure of most of the victims was apparently minimal. Nevertheless, it caused skin damage that scientists described as looking remarkably like the skin damage caused by overexposure to x-rays. After a long investigation, the new chemical was cautiously applied to see if it might have the same effect as x-rays on cancer. To a considerable degree, it did.

From this odd discovery came the development of what are now known as cytotoxic or immunosuppressive drugs.* They are administered today by cancer specialists in the treatment of certain types of cancer, usually in cases that cannot be helped by surgery. Because they act to suppress the body's normal immune mechanisms, they are also employed in organ transplantation to keep the body from rejecting what it identifies as a foreign body. And, because deranged immune reactions are seemingly involved in certain forms of arthritis, the immunosuppressives are now being cautiously tested in carefully selected patients who have the most serious forms of the disease.

Experts emphasize that the known toxicity of these agents is so high that their use should be restricted to life-threatening situations, as in treating lupus complicated by serious kidney disease, or in treating seriously crippling rheumatoid arthritis that has failed to respond to more conventional therapy, or when a patient cannot tolerate less hazardous drugs. Before starting immunosuppressive treatment, a physician usually recommends consultation with an expert, and a patient undergoing such treatment should be followed with the greatest care. The treatment should be terminated as soon as possible.

Levamisole. An odd addition to this list of experimental drugs for the treatment of arthritis is, of all things, a remedy for roundworm, hookworm, and other nematodes that can invade the gastrointestinal tract. Introduced in 1965 by a Belgian firm, Janssen Pharmaceutica, it is used in many countries in treating both human beings and animals. In the

---

* Among the products in this family are chlorambucil, marketed under the brand name of Leukeran, and azathioprine, marketed under the brand name of Imuran, both by Burroughs Wellcome; cyclophosphamide, marketed under the brand name of Cytoxan by Mead Johnson; and methotrexate, marketed by Lederle.

United States, is has thus far been approved by the FDA for only veterinary use.

Levamisole* has one other characteristic. Not only does it help to kill worms, but, unlike the immunosuppressive drugs, it also steps up the body's immune defense mechanisms.

In 1974, several of us at the University of California, San Francisco, decided to test it in rheumatoid arthritis. This decision was not based on a blind guess. There were a few scattered clues from the work of early bacteriologists who found that injections of an antituberculosis vaccine— impractical for long-term use—not only enhanced immune reactions, but might have had a slightly beneficial effect in arthritis.

With the discovery of the new Belgian product, we had an immunity-stimulating drug that could be used for long periods. Its major side effects seemed to be a decrease in the white blood cell count (a serious possibility that requires periodic checking) and a skin rash. These effects could be minimized by using smaller doses.

By 1978, the UCSF group had tested levamisole under the controls required by the FDA on about a hundred victims of rheumatoid arthritis. In all of them, the disease could no longer be controlled by any of the standard antiarthritis drugs, including gold salts, or by anything except dangerously large amounts of corticosteroid hormones.

Like gold salts, the new drug is slow to take effect, and no change was apparent in our patients for at least three or four months. After that time, however, there was marked improvement in at least half of the patients, many of whom have continued to improve significantly.

The long-term results on larger groups of patients are yet to be determined. Our colleagues elsewhere in the United States and in Europe are now conducting their own studies.

Even the preliminary success achieved with this immunity-enhancing chemical has given some tentative support to the century-old notion that rheumatoid arthritis may be, after all, an infectious disease, possibly caused by a slow-acting and yet-to-be detected virus.

* Marketed as levamisole by Janssen Research and Development in the United States exclusively for use on animals.

The Drugs Against Gout

For gout, which is marked by excessive amounts of uric acid salts in the blood and urate deposits in the joints, kidneys, and other parts of the body, aspirin—the accepted remedy for other forms of arthritis—has been used, sometimes with beneficial results. If the aspirin is administered in large doses, it may help to remove uric acid through the kidneys. In small quantities, however, it may reduce the excretion of uric acid. In addition, it is now recognized that, if aspirin and one of the modern gout-preventive drugs are given simultaneously, the therapeutic action of the latter may be nullified, and an attack may be triggered.

As noted earlier in this chapter, such accepted anti-inflammatory agents as phenylbutazone and indomethacin have proved valuable in acute attacks of gout.

Recently, it has been reported that at least some of the newer nonsteroidal anti-inflammatory agents most commonly administered in rheumatoid arthritis may also be helpful in controlling an acute attack of gout.

Colchicine. In ancient times in the region of Colchis in Asia Minor, the home of Medea and the place where Jason sought the Golden Fleece, there grew a plant now called *Colchicum autumnale,* commonly meadow saffron or autumn crocus. At first it was highly regarded as a source of poison and later as a valuable medicine. (Many other useful drug products, including a number of remedies for heart disease, likewise began with an evil reputation.) As early as the sixth century A.D., it was recommended for the treatment of joint pain in

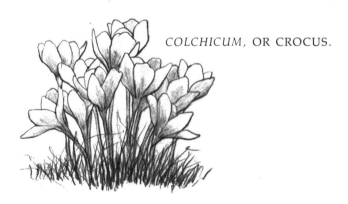

COLCHICUM, OR CROCUS.

general, and in 1763 it was proposed specifically for gout, by Baron Anton von Störk. In 1820, two remarkable French scientists, Pierre Pelletier and Joseph Caventou, developed a simple procedure to extract alkaloids from their crude plant sources. In that year, they isolated quinine from cinchona bark and, in the same year, they isolated from *Colchicum* the active ingredient that they named colchicine.

In the century and a half since then, colchicine has been the primary drug for the treatment of an acute attack of gout. Even now, the mechanism of its action is not completely understood. It has no significant effect on the amount of uric acid in the body or on urate excretion by the kidneys. The drug seems to act simply by countering the gouty inflammation.

Although newer drugs have been synthesized that prevent acute attacks, either by accelerating the excretion of urate salts or by inhibiting their formation in the body, colchicine is still prescribed in small doses as a preventive, especially if the patient is plagued with frequently recurring attacks.

Adverse reactions to large doses include nausea, vomiting, and diarrhea. In many cases, these reactions can be avoided by the use of lower dosages.

Probenecid. If scientists at Sharp & Dohme—later to be merged with Merck—had started out to develop a drug to control gout, probenecid* might never have been discovered. What started these investigators was the vexing fact that, in the early 1940s, penicillin was too scarce, too difficult to produce, and too expensive. Complicating the situation was the additional fact that penicillin was excreted rapidly by the kidneys. In the first human subject treated with penicillin, an Oxford policeman, Oxford University scientists attempted to deal with the problem by collecting all the patient's urine, concentrating it, taking out and purifying the penicillin, and re-injecting the antibiotic time after time into the policeman. Tragically, though he showed dramatic improvement for a few days, the supply of penicillin ran out and he died.

---

* Marketed under the brand name of Benemid by Merck Sharp & Dohme and under the generic name of probenecid by other companies.

Starting in 1943, the Sharp & Dohme team sought a drug that would slow down penicillin excretion. The first product they found decreased the loss of penicillin, but it, too, was excreted so rapidly from the body that the patient needed to take it in quantities of about half a pound per day. Soon a second compound was synthesized that was somewhat better; it was effective in a daily dosage of approximately half an ounce.

In their investigations, the scientists did not study only drugs. They uncovered remarkable new information about the many and complicated secretory mechanisms of the kidneys, and the ways in which these mechanisms could be affected by drugs. This basic research led in 1947 to the synthesis of probenecid, which in very small doses effectively controlled the loss of penicillin.

Sadly, it seemed, the discovery had come too late. Penicillin was no longer so expensive and difficult to produce. Furthermore, several groups had produced penicillin derivatives that remain in the body long enough to control infections.

"Although it looked as though probenecid was a commercial failure," a Sharp & Dohme official said later, "we continued our studies. And then we found that while it decreased the excretion of some substances, probenecid increased the excretion of others—including uric acid. We suddenly discovered we had a potential remedy for gout."

Clinical tests soon demonstrated that the agent had remarkable value, not in controlling an acute attack of gout, but in preventing attacks by lowering the level of uric acid in the blood. The drug was first marketed for gout therapy in 1952.

Experts warn that probenecid should be administered with caution to any patient having a history of uric acid stones in the kidneys or other kidney disease.

Sulfinpyrazone.   In the 1950s, with evidence of the value of phenylbutazone in treating a number of forms of arthritis, especially gout, the Geigy scientists in Switzerland prepared a variety of phenylbutazone derivatives in the hope that at least one of them would be even more useful. A series of these derivatives was sent for testing to various scientists, including a group of investigators at the National Heart Institute and several cooperating hospitals in New York City.

One of the new compounds, bearing the code name of G-25671, turned out to be substantially though not sensationally better than phenylbutazone. Its mechanism of action, however, was far different. Instead of controlling inflammation, G-25671 helped the body flush out excessive quantities of uric acid through the urine. Tests in human subjects also showed that, when G-25671 was broken down in the body, it was transformed into a different compound, now known as sulfinpyrazone.* Its action as a uricosuric agent in flushing out uric acid was remarkable.

In their report submitted for publication in 1956, the team of scientists headed by Dr. John J. Burns of the National Heart Institute said that their preliminary studies suggested that "it is the most potent uricosuric agent yet described." Within two years, tests in Great Britain and the United States showed that sulfinpyrazone was clearly effective against gout in human subjects.

Like other antigout drugs, this one can cause side effects in some patients, but they are reported to be relatively minor and uncommon. Nevertheless, especially if sulfinpyrazone is to be used for prolonged periods, repeated blood tests are usually recommended. Caution is also indicated if there is a record of uric acid kidney stones.

Allopurinol. One way to find a new or better drug is to synthesize a hundred, or a thousand, or perhaps ten thousand more or less related compounds that might possibly work, and then screen them in the hope that one or two of the chemicals will be useful.

Another is to attempt to decipher the underlying chemistry of a disease process and then, on the basis of such knowledge, to hand-tailor a few substances that might block the unwanted process.

Among the most elegant examples of the second approach is the development of allopurinol† and its introduction for the treatment of gout. Under the direction of Dr. George Hitchings of Burroughs Wellcome, it became a twenty-five-year project undertaken without any clear idea at the start of what practical results it might yield. What it

* Marketed by Ciba-Geigy under the brand name of Anturane.
† Marketed under the brand name of Zyloprim by Burroughs Wellcome.

117

did yield was not merely a fascinating view—fascinating at least to scientists—of how the body works, but also highly practical new agents for the treatment of a number of forms of leukemia, bacterial infections, malaria, and gout, and substances to increase the success of organ transplants.

Starting with a study of the nucleic acids—then thought to be rather unexciting substances, in the days before DNA, RNA, and the genetic code became of worldwide interest— the Burroughs Wellcome research eventually came upon a new drug called 6-mercaptopurine, or 6-MP. In early trials, 6-MP worked against leukemia, but only up to a point. In the body, it was speedily changed and degraded by an enzyme called xanthine oxidase. This enzyme was no stranger to biochemists, who knew that it played a role in the metabolism of purines. The trick, then, was to find a way to inhibit or block the action of the enzyme so that more of the 6-MP would remain in the body and keep active against the leukemia.

The scientists had done their homework on xanthine oxidase. They were aware that the enzyme could be blocked by specially constructed chemicals. One of these was allopurinol. Tests disclosed that allopurinol was well tolerated by the body and that it increased the effectiveness of 6-MP.

The investigators were also aware that xanthine oxidase was involved in more than flushing out 6-MP. The enzyme also played a key role in transforming purines eventually into uric acid, the chemical villain in gout. The value of allopurinol in gout was demonstrated clinically in the mid-1960s.

Unlike other antigout remedies, allopurinol has no value in stepping up the excretion of uric acid through the kidneys. Rather, it limits the production of uric acid in the first place.

In gout patients, allopurinol is no remedy for an acute attack. Instead, it is used after such an attack has subsided in order to prevent the accumulation of uric acid and its salts in the body, thus preventing a new attack.

Like other antigout and antiarthritis drugs, allopurinol can produce unpleasant or even dangerous side effects. Generally, the side effects are so uncommon that most gout patients can take the drug comfortably for many years, and perhaps indefinitely.

How Do They Work?

The mechanism of action of antiarthritis agents, except some of the drugs used against gout, has long been a mystery. Scientists still do not know how these substances work against inflammation in the joints, or in any other parts of the body.

Now exciting the interest of drug experts is the possible role played by a group of hormonelike regulators known as prostaglandins. Originally, it was believed that they were produced by the prostate gland—hence their name. It is now known that they are produced in many parts of the body.

As a result of long years of basic research conducted in Great Britain, Sweden, The Netherlands, and notably by Upjohn in the United States, investigators have found that the prostaglandins somehow affect the stomach, the intestines, the reproductive system, the heart, the kidneys, the lungs, and the blood system.

In the early 1970s, British scientists found that the prostaglandins are involved in *causing* pain, fever, and inflammation. Aspirin and its relatives seem to work by limiting the formation of these hormonelike substances.

Whether this is the solution to the whole puzzle or, more likely, only one piece of it remains to be ascertained. Nevertheless, knowledge of the role of prostaglandins in inducing inflammation may help investigators discover new and better antiarthritis drugs in the future. Moreover, research in this field may eventually cast light on what causes the disease in the first place.

Drug-Drug Interactions

Modern pharmacologists—the physicians or scientists who are the experts on drugs—are well aware that many widely used drugs can interact with each other or with certain foods. Some of these interactions can be beneficial, but others can be dangerous.

Among the drugs used in treating arthritis, for example, the action of indomethacin can be undesirably increased if the patient is simultaneously using probenecid to control gout. The effect of the corticosteroids can be inhibited if the patient is also taking antiepilepsy drugs or phenobarbital. Many of the immunosuppressive agents can react dangerously with the corticosteroids and gout remedies. Aspirin and some of the other antiarthritis agents can react with anticoagulants to cause serious hemorrhage and with oral antidiabetic drugs to cause shock.

In many instances, these difficulties can be corrected simply by adjusting the dosages. In any case, the prescribing physician must be aware of *all* the drugs being used simultaneously by the patient.

The Matter of Drug Costs

The prices charged for both prescription drugs and over-the-counter preparations, including those commonly used in the treatment of arthritis, have been the subject of increasing attention since 1958, when the late Senator Estes Kefauver began his hearings on the drug industry. Further attention was focused on the problem as the result of hearings chaired by Senator Gaylord Nelson in the late 1960s and the 1970s and studies by a special task force in the U.S. Department of Health, Education, and Welfare.

From these and other investigations, certain points stand out:

Drug prices have increased substantially in the past few decades, but by no means as rapidly as hospital and physician charges.

In general, the pharmaceutical industry has made sizeable net profits year after year. Any drastic reduction in this profit rate, however, could threaten the willingness of the industry to support new research needed for the development of new and better drugs.

In most, though not all, cases, the price of a particular drug is lowered after the seventeen-year patent on it expires, and it can be marketed by competitors under its generic name rather than under its original brand name.

There are increasing efforts to lower drug expenditures by requiring pharmacies to post the retail prices of the drugs they dispense, and by allowing or requiring pharmacists to substi-

tute a low-cost version for the more expensive brand-name
drug actually prescribed by the physician. It is not yet clear
what effect these moves will have on drug expenditures
under specific third-party drug insurance programs such as
those included in Medicare, Medicaid, Blue Cross/Blue
Shield, private health programs, and union health plans.
Most prescription drugs now on the market are still under
patent, and no generic versions are legally available.
With extremely few exceptions in recent years, there is no evidence
to show that there is any significant difference in quality between formulations, brand or generic, of the same active ingredients. These exceptions have been more notorious than
numerous. In some, both the brand-name and the generic-
name drugs are produced by the same manufacturer.

The importance of drug costs to a patient may depend
on whether the drug is needed for a short-term acute illness
or for long-term therapy for a chronic disease. Thus, the high
cost of an antibiotic prescribed for perhaps ten days in the
treatment of an infection like pneumonia may be less painful
financially than that of an antiasthma or antiarthritis drug
that is needed for many months or years. For a drug required
to combat an acute infection, most patients will go to the
nearest pharmacy, regardless of prices. For an antiarthritis
drug, prudent patients will shop around and compare prices
and, if the patient is truly prudent, the services offered by
various pharmacies.

The table beginning on page 122 gives the monthly
cost of the drugs most commonly used in treating arthritis
(with the exception of gold salts). The figures given are aver-
ages of prices charged *at the retail level* by a number of independent pharmacies and chain store pharmacies in the same
area at the same time in late 1978. In some cases, chain store
prices were lower but, in others, the prices in chain pharmacies were the same or higher. The prices given in the table are
for purchases of 100 units—capsules or tablets—although
physicians may prescribe a drug in larger or smaller quantities. Ordinarily, the price per unit is less if the quantity
ordered is large.

The daily dosages shown here are those generally prescribed by many rheumatologists. However, on the basis of
their own experience, physicians may prescribe differently.

It must be emphasized that the goal of rational prescribing is not to save money. Rational prescribing means select-

121

MONTHLY RETAIL COSTS OF ORAL ARTHRITIS DRUGS

Based on a far-from-complete survey conducted late in 1978 in the San Francisco area, covering both independent pharmacies and chain stores, the prices in this table are for purchases of 100 units—that is, 100 capsules or 100 tablets. They will undoubtedly be different in different parts of the country, and will vary depending on the daily dosage recommended for a particular patient.

Drug	Weight per unit (mg)	Usual daily dosage (mg)	Retail cost per 100 units	Usual cost per month
OVER-THE-COUNTER PRODUCTS	(a)	(b)		
Generic aspirin			$ 0.60	$ 1.44– 3.60
Bayer Aspirin			1.54	3.70– 9.24
Generic buffered aspirin			1.50	3.60– 9.00
Bufferin			2.59	6.22–15.54
Anacin	(c)	(d)	2.62	5.03–12.58
NONSTEROIDS				
Phenylbutazone				
Ciba-Geigy: Butazolidin	100	100–300	13.33	4.00–12.00
Generic phenylbutazone	100	100–300	11.50	3.45–10.35
Indomethacin	25	50–150	18.00	6.85–32.40
Merck Sharp & Dohme: Indocin	50		22.83	
Hydroxychloroquine				
Winthrop: Plaquenil	200	200	18.36	5.51
Penicillamine				
Merck Sharp & Dohme: Cuprimine	250	250–1,000	29.00	8.70–34.80
Ibuprofen	300	1,200–1,600	15.00	18.00–20.04
Upjohn: Motrin	400		16.00	
Fenoprofen				
Lilly: Nalfon	600	2,400	20.00	24.00
Naproxen				
Syntex: Naprosyn	250	500–750	26.14	15.68–23.52
Tolmetin				
McNeil: Tolectin	400	1,200	15.86	28.54
Sulindac	150	300–400	31.00	18.60–22.20
Merck Sharp & Dohme: Clinoril	200		37.00	
CORTICOSTEROID HORMONES (e)				
Cortisone (generic)	25	25–75	9.86	2.96– 8.88
Hydrocortisone (generic)	20	20–60	16.44	4.93–14.79
Prednisone (generic)	5	5–15	5.50	1.65– 4.95

MONTHLY RETAIL COSTS OF ORAL ARTHRITIS DRUGS
(Continued)

Drug	Weight per unit (mg)	Usual daily dosage (mg)	Retail cost per 100 units	Usual cost per month
Betamethasone				
Schering: Celestone	0.6	0.6–1.8	22.82	6.85–20.55
Triamcinolone				
Lederle: Aristocort	4	4–12	27.10	8.13–24.39
Methylprednisolone				
Upjohn: Medrol	4	4–12	26.81	8.04–24.12
ANTIGOUT DRUGS				
Colchicine (generic)	0.5	0.5–1.0(f)	8.60	2.58–5.16
Probenecid				
Merck Sharp & Dohme: Benemid	500	1,000–2,000	11.96	7.18–15.48
Generic probenecid	500	1,000–2,000	9.75	5.85–11.70
Sulfinpyrazone				
Ciba-Geigy: Anturane	200	200–400	16.16	4.85– 9.70
Allopurinol				
Burroughs Wellcome: Zyloprim	100	200–400	11.80	7.08–14.16

[a] All aspirin products listed except Anacin contain 5 grains of aspirin per tablet.

[b] All except Anacin may be prescribed in quantities of 8 to 20 tablets per day.

[c] Anacin contains $6\frac{2}{3}$ grains of aspirin per tablet.

[d] May be prescribed in quantities of 6 to 16 tablets per day.

[e] Infrequently, as in serious cases of lupus, these hormones may be prescribed in quantities as much as four times the usual amount, which would make drug costs as high as $96.00 per month.

[f] This is the dosage range usually employed for prevention. In an acute attack, a dose of 3.0 to 6.0 mg daily may be prescribed for a few days.

ing the right drug for the right patient, at the right time and in the right amounts. Reducing costs is important, and cannot be ignored, but it is not as critical as achieving the best possible clinical results.

In recent years, many drug experts have been urging patients to request their physicians to prescribe generically or to ask pharmacists to substitute a lower-priced product if one is on the market and if substitution is permitted under existing laws. In 1978, drug product substitution was allowed or required in about forty states in the United States. In most states, if a physician has no confidence in the quality or acceptability of a particular generic product for a particular patient, he or she can instruct the pharmacist *not* to make a substitution.

We feel it important to emphasize that, regardless of the claims of some companies, the use of generic products does not represent second-class drug therapy. The overall quality of generic-name drugs is high, and their use may afford significant savings to patients or their third-party carriers. Patients should never hesitate to take up the subject with their physicians and pharmacists.

CHAPTER 12

ARTHRITIS SURGERY

Attempts to repair the damage of arthritis by surgical operations are presumably as old as surgery itself. Until the latter part of the nineteenth century, the results probably ranked between poor and gruesome.

One problem was the ever-present threat of infection. Until the introduction of antiseptic surgery in the 1860s and the use of aseptic surgical methods after that, infection was frighteningly common. Even in a relatively simple procedure, the amputation of a limb, death rates of 20 percent were reported a century ago in Massachusetts, 43 percent in Edinburgh, 46 percent in Zurich, and 60 percent in Paris. Joseph Lister's use of carbolic acid, first tried on a surgical patient in 1865, showed dramatically how these percentages could be reduced. Further advances came with the application of aseptic methods—aimed at preventing infection in the first place—and then with the use of constantly improved antibacterial agents and finally with the antibiotics.

An equally serious problem was the lack of an effective means for controlling pain. One surgeon commented: "You made your man drunk, and the porters and students held him down, and you had to set your teeth and finish the job fast." In the early 1800s, the good surgeon was the quick surgeon. Operations that are now scheduled for two or three hours were completed from first incision to last stitch in seven minutes. All this changed almost miraculously with the first general anesthetics that came into use in the late 1840s. Since then, anesthesia has become increasingly safe, smooth, and effective.

In some surgical procedures, cutting into blood vessels was inevitable, and severe hemorrhage was once a major problem. Now, with blood transfusions being simple, safe, and relatively inexpensive, loss of blood in the course of an operation is no longer a matter of great concern.

Finally, in the past, the surgery itself was considered to be the only thing that counted. Once the operation had been completed, if the patients survived, they were on their own. The complex physical and emotional problems of convalescence were deemed to be of little or no importance. Now recovery from arthritis surgery is looked upon as being almost as important as the surgery itself. Most patients are prepared in advance with carefully planned programs to cope with the often difficult stresses that must be faced for weeks or sometimes months before there is a return to normal activity.

Today, the surgeon may enter into the act many weeks—perhaps as much as six months—before any surgery is scheduled. The surgeon gets to know the patient, the patient's clinical condition, the patient's living arrangements, and the patient's hopes, fears, and financial situation, including insurance coverage.

In taking this approach, it is invaluable to recruit the patient's family physician or rheumatologist, the surgeon, and often a physical therapist, sometimes well before the surgery is started.

The results of all these developments have been gratifying in most cases. They will be even better in the future. Arthritis surgery—once considered a drastic, risky, last-ditch procedure to be contemplated only when all else has failed—has become an accepted part of arthritis treatment.

When is surgery indicated? The major indication in most cases is not crippling or joint deformity but intractable pain—pain that cannot be satisfactorily controlled by drugs, rest, exercise, and applications of heat or cold. When the pain becomes so severe that the patients are unable to take care of themselves, perform the minimum of essential duties at home or work, or sleep at night, the time may have come for surgery.

An operation may also be considered in those cases in which deformity and disability have resulted from a muscular contraction, of the type, for example, that makes it impossible for the patient to straighten a knee and to stand upright. The pain might not be severe; a simple surgical operation, however, can restore nearly complete function and is often performed mainly for this purpose.

Referrals and the Second Opinion

The job of the orthopedic surgeon is more than doing the technical operation. It also includes deciding which patient is likely to benefit from the operation, when it should be performed (in a month, three months, six months, or longer), and which procedure is preferred. As with many other aspects of medicine, the ability to make these judgments is rarely learned in medical school. It takes the experience acquired only after long training under the tutelage of an already-experienced expert, and then years of practice.

It is our hope that, except in an emergency, no one but a skilled orthopedic surgeon would be willing to undertake the surgical treatment of arthritis nowadays. And, for arthritis, emergency surgery is uncommon.

Probably all family physicians, internists, pediatricians, rheumatologists, and even general surgeons—those well able to perform abdominal surgery, repair broken bones, and the like—are well aware that operations on the joints require special competence. Among orthopedic surgeons themselves, there are those who feel able to do a total replacement of the hip but will not undertake the more formidable replacement of the knee joint. Surgeons recognize that joint surgery may require special facilities and equipment that are not available in every hospital.

Ordinarily, when, for example, a family physician thinks that a patient's arthritis is getting out of control and it may be necessary to turn from relatively harmless drugs to more potent but more hazardous agents, consultation with a rheumatologist may be desirable. Consideration of surgery should call for consultation and what is known as the second opinion. For this second view, advice should be sought from an arthritis specialist or rheumatologist, or an orthopedic surgeon with particular experience in the treatment of arthritis, or both. Such consultation is now being required more and more frequently under a number of insurance programs.

Rarely is speed required. Most experienced arthritis surgeons feel the long-term outcome will be most successful when they can have ample time to analyze the situation and

129

plan for both surgery and convalescence. In these early stages, certain guidelines should be known to the patient:

Beware the physician who responds to a suggestion for a second opinion or a referral by asking, "Why? Don't you trust me?"

The answer to such a question should be a temperate "No!"

It is our experience that most physicians, unless they feel unsure of themselves, welcome the opportunity of getting expert advice. In the same way, most patients seem to have greater respect for a physician who recognizes his own limitations and is perfectly willing to call for help.

Beware the surgeon who sees a patient for the first time on one day and schedules surgery for the next.

Except under unusual circumstances, experienced orthopedic surgeons will want to learn as much as possible about the patient. Does the patient live alone or with someone who can provide help during the difficult days after discharge from the hospital? Does the patient live on one floor, or are there stairs to be climbed? What will happen emotionally and financially if the patient does not return to full-time employment for four weeks, or eight weeks, or twelve weeks? If there are young children in the family, who will take care of them? How much does the patient smoke? (Involved here is lung function and minimizing the risk of postsurgical pneumonia or other lung problem.) Is the patient overweight, and can the excess be reduced before surgery? (Postsurgical complications such as inflammation of the leg veins and possibly infection are more likely to occur in obese patients.) What is the patient's tolerance for pain? For the amount of damage revealed by examination, is the pain more or less than what might be expected?

Beware the surgeon who urges or induces a patient to undergo surgery.

Most competent surgeons will explain as completely and simply as possible what the situation is—what will be done, what results might be normally expected, what complications there might be and what risks must be faced, what problems should be expected during convalescence, and what lifestyle limitations—if any—there will be. On the basis of this knowledge, and any additional information

gained from consultation, it is the patient's responsibility to
say "yea" or "nay."

Sitting down beforehand with the patient and discus-
sing such matters is not done simply to avert a possible mal-
practice suit if something goes wrong. Physicians are generally aware that a fully informed patient is more likely to do
well under treatment, and the outcome will probably be
better.

The Matter of Costs

Whether or not current health care costs are low, reasonable,
or outrageously high may be a controversial subject, but it
can scarcely come as a surprise to most Americans that doctor bills and hospital charges are at all-time highs and still
rising. Patients contemplating surgery and the necessary
hospitalization must consider such matters unless they have
essentially full-coverage health insurance or unusually large
financial assets, or are immune to emotional trauma.

It is probably impossible to give a realistic estimate of
the nationwide costs for arthritis hospitalization and surgery. They vary greatly in different parts of the United
States. They may even vary among specialists and among
hospitals in the same area. The fees that a doctor charges
may vary as well, depending on whether the patient has
health insurance and, if so, what kind. If there are complications at the outset, or if they occur during or after the operation, more care will be needed and costs will almost certainly
be higher.

For several of the important surgical procedures discussed in the following sections, relative prices are indicated. It should be emphasized that these figures are derived
from late-1978 costs in an area in which the cost of medical
care is usually considered to be among the highest in the
United States. In most other parts of the country, the figures
were probably lower. In a few, they were higher.

The total cost of any given operation reported here includes three main items: the surgeon's fee; the room-and-
board charge made by the hospital; and a group of expenses
including charges for the operating room, laboratory services, x-rays, blood transfusions and drugs, the cost of

whatever metallic or plastic replacement may be inserted, the anesthetic, and the anesthetist's fee. Where it is possible and permissible, some thoughtful surgeons will have much of the testing performed before the patient is admitted so that the number of days of expensive hospitalization can be kept to a minimum.

For patients covered under existing Medicare regulations in 1978—usually those of age sixty-five or older—the program was paying 80 percent of all costs, less a relatively small deductible. The hospital or the surgeon could accept the Medicare payment as reimbursement in full or ask the patient to pay the remaining 20 percent.

Under the provisions of Medicaid, designed primarily for people having low incomes, the payment covered approximately 60 percent of the total cost, depending on the program in each state. A physician or hospital accepting a Medicaid patient had to agree in advance to accept the Medicaid payment as reimbursement in full.

Nongovernmental health insurance—including policies written by Blue Cross/Blue Shield and private insurance programs—differed widely. Patients should find out for themselves what current coverage they have.

If it is necessary to plan on care for weeks or months in a nursing home after hospitalization, or to arrange for home health care, physical therapy, occupational rehabilitation, or psychological support, patients should determine what coverage—if any—that they have for such services.

Getting such information in advance is not always as easy as it should be. Probably the best place to start is with the surgeon. The day has long since passed when discussion of dollars and cents was considered to be tactless or indelicate. Now most doctors prefer to get this matter out on the table at the start, certainly long before the patient expresses shock or outrage at the size of the bill. Today most physicians maintain what they call a schedule of "usual, customary, and necessary" fees that they charge all patients, all Medicare and Medicaid programs, and all private insurance companies except those that work on their own fee schedules. Patients who have financial problems may be surprised but pleased to discover that physicians are often willing to adjust their fees downward or make arrangements for a mutually satisfactory payment schedule. It is usually far better to make these arrangements in advance rather than after the bills have been mailed.

Experienced surgeons are also usually able to estimate the length of the operation (which determines in part the cost of the operating room) and the probable length of hospitalization. In this connection, it is important to note that most modern orthopedic surgeons do not favor needlessly prolonged hospital stays; they want the patients discharged from the hospital and sent home as quickly as possible.

(All the foregoing, obviously, is based on the present system—or nonsystem—of health insurance. If a broad program of national health insurance is put into effect— probably not before 1984 or 1985 at the earliest—things may be different.)

Synovectomies

In rheumatoid arthritis, it has long been recognized that the trouble seems to be centered in the synovial membrane, the inner lining of the joint, which becomes thickened, inflamed, and painful. For more than half a century, surgeons have attempted to alleviate the symptoms and prevent progressive destruction of the joint cartilage by simply removing this inner lining in a procedure known as a synovectomy. In the past, this operation was usually performed on only one joint, less often on several, and only when there was intractable pain. Most commonly involved were joints in the knee, the wrist, or the fingers.

Most patients recovered from the surgery with marked or even dramatic relief of symptoms. Pain was strikingly controlled, and motion of the joint became easier although occasionally somewhat restricted. Unfortunately, it was found, the synovial membrane frequently grew back in a few years, became inflamed again, and the symptoms returned.

Synovectomies are still being done today, although they are performed less frequently, having been replaced by other procedures. The operation itself may take from one to two hours, and the patient is hospitalized for perhaps five to seven days. If the operation is performed on a wrist or finger joint, it may be necessary for the patient to wear a temporary brace or splint after surgery. Full use of the joint may require from six weeks to several months. After a knee synovectomy, temporary support is usually required for one to three

133

weeks, and adequate use of the joint may not be possible for four to eight weeks.

In the high-cost area surveyed here, the surgeon's fee may be about $1,400, the hospital room-and-board charges about $1,100, and the other charges roughly $1,500.

Joint Fusion

Some victims of rheumatoid arthritis or osteoarthritis have uncontrollable pain in one joint but only when the joint is moved. For many decades, an accepted procedure for solving the problem has been to prevent motion by fusing the bones together, a procedure called arthrodesis. It was once performed on virtually any joint but is now used most frequently on the wrist, the fingers, the ankle, the toes, and the top vertebrae in the neck. For other joints, surgeons are turning more and more often to the insertion of a joint replacement. For some patients, except those having rheumatoid arthritis, surgeons may still elect fusion to immobilize a hip or knee.

Operating time may be from one to four hours, depending on the joint. The basic procedure is to get at the ends of the two bones meeting in the joint, remove the damaged cartilage, cut down to expose the healthy bone ends, and press these tightly together. The pressure is sometimes maintained by pins that go through each bone and extend outside the body; by means of two screw clamps attached to the pins, the bones can be held together until fusion is complete. The pins are removed quickly in a second operation.

About fourteen days of hospitalization is normally necessary for fusion of the knee joint. Fusion is usually complete within three to six months.

If surgery performed on the hip or knee results in shortening of the limb, it is generally shorter by not more than about a centimeter, or three-eights of an inch. The difference can be corrected by wearing a special shoe lift.

The surgical fee customarily runs to about $1,500, the hospital room-and-board charge to $2,500, and other hospital charges to about $2,250.

Tendon Repair

One of the more unpleasant complications of rheumatoid arthritis may come on suddenly and call for immediate attention. Usually affecting tendons in the wrist, the disease process can destroy the tendon or turn the slick outer surface of the bone into a rough surface that will fray the tendon sheath and eventually tear it. The result may be an inability to use one or more fingers.

Depending on the circumstances, the surgeon may elect to use one of several different procedures, removing the damaged bone surface, repairing the torn tissues, and sometimes attaching the weakened tendon to another healthy tendon alongside it. The procedure generally takes from one to two hours, with three or four days of hospitalization necessary. Adequate use of the wrist becomes possible in about two to four months.

The surgeon may charge from $300 to $700 for a tendon repair, the hospital room-and-board bill will be about $600, and miscellaneous hospital charges will be roughly $1,250.

Total Replacement of the Hip

Perhaps the most devastatingly crippling form of arthritis is that attacking the hip. The pain and stiffness can be so severe that walking is impossible, and the patient can barely move from wheelchair to bed. Some victims are totally bedridden. Some cannot get adequate care at home and must be resigned to spending the rest of their lives in a nursing home.

Anatomists and orthopedic surgeons have long held the opinion that a hip destroyed by arthritis is theoretically well suited for an artificial replacement, or prosthesis. Unlike other joints, the hip is well protected by thick layers of muscle and connective tissue. The socket of the joint is firmly seated in the pelvis. The ball is part of the thigh bone, one of the largest and strongest in the body. Thus, it should be a technically simple procedure to substitute artificial devices for the ball and the socket. But, when daring surgeons attempted to do so, they encountered three seemingly in-

135

surmountable hurdles: first, the body reacted to any substitute material then available as if it were a foreign body, producing severe inflammation and tissue destruction; second, the replacement itself eroded or rusted and often broke; and third, whether the replacement were screwed or glued into place, it sooner or later—and usually sooner—came loose and had to be removed.

As early as 1938, surgeons were attempting total hip replacement on a few selected patients. These were desperation measures, and practically all failed. Some of the patients later required amputation, and some died because of complications. Nevertheless, a few patients agreed to undergo this last-ditch procedure, probably because they felt their life was already hopeless.

Since then, as a result of pioneering efforts in Great Britain, the United States, and other countries, the surgical techniques have been improved. The use of special stainless steels helped to reduce tissue reaction, as did that of a cobalt-chromium-molybdenum alloy that was highly resistant to wear and essentially inert in the body. With the advent of tough, wear-resistant plastics that could be highly polished, prospects were even better.

Much of the credit for developing what is now the most widely used total hip replacement is given to John Charnley, a British surgeon, and his associates at the Centre for Hip Surgery at Wrightington Hospital in the small town of Wiggin, Lancashire. Long an internationally recognized authority on orthopedics and author of a standard textbook on the treatment of fractures, Charnley combined the three ingredients that spelled success: a highly polished cup made of polyethylene plastic to replace the damaged socket in the pelvis; a highly polished metal replacement for the ball, which has a long, tapering stem to fit snugly into the shaft of the thigh bone; and a methyl methacrylate cement to hold the replacements in place.

The two replacements must be carefully selected for each patient, and detailed x-ray studies are essential to determine the precise dimensions that will be needed.

Orthopedists estimate that the operation is now being performed on about 80,000 patients a year—many of them in their seventies or eighties—in the United States alone, with a rate of success of about 95 percent. In a few instances, the joint may be attacked by a new or a long-slumbering infec-

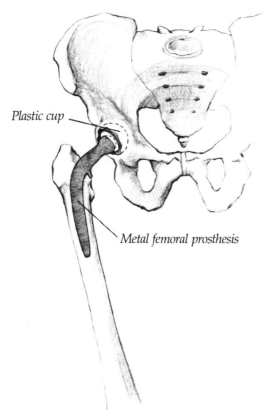

HIP PROSTHESIS

Plastic cup

Metal femoral prosthesis

TOTAL
REPLACEMENT OF
THE HIP JOINT.

tion. The replacement in the thigh bone may break, and a second operation is required for the installation of another. Many of the first patients treated in England fifteen years ago are reported to be alive and well, with virtually no disability.

Patients scheduled for total hip replacement are generally admitted to the hospital from one to four days before surgery for the necessary tests to be completed. The operation itself includes reaming out the socket in the pelvis, removing the end of the thigh bone, applying the cementing ingredients—which are quickly hardened through a heat-generating process—and then inserting and adjusting the replacements. The operation itself customarily requires from two to three hours, although it may take longer.

Some surgeons have their patients standing beside their beds on the third or fourth day after surgery and leaving the hospital, walking with the assistance of crutches, within two or three weeks. Others start the action more promptly.

"We usually have the patient standing by the bed on the day after surgery," one orthopedist says. "This may cause some additional pain, and we don't try to prevent it with morphine. The pain will make the patient take deeper and faster breaths, and that will improve lung action. On the average, our patients will remain in the hospital for about fourteen days, but this can vary tremendously. We tell them that when you can get in and out of bed by yourself, on and off the toilet by yourself, in and out of a chair by yourself, and manage a flight of stairs, you're ready to go home. Some are out of the hospital in eight days."

In many cases, patients can walk without crutches and return to work in about four to six weeks, although this may vary with the age and general health of the patient and the nature of the work. Usually, heavy manual labor is prohibited, and such activities as running, jogging, and jumping are barred forever.

For an ordinary uncomplicated hip replacement, the surgeon's fee may be from $2,100 to $2,500, the hospitalization cost is about $2,500, and the other charges range from approximately $2,000 to $3,000. The replacement itself may cost $600 or more.

Special problems, and sometimes additional costs, may be encountered in doing a hip replacement in a child or in a patient suffering from softening of the bone.

Total Replacement of the Knee

A more recent procedure than the hip operation, total replacement of the knee now seems to be out of the category of experimental procedures. About 30,000 knee replacements are performed annually in this country. These are somewhat trickier, and some surgeons who feel they are competent to undertake a hip replacement will refer a knee replacement to a specially experienced colleague. In comparison with the hip, the knee is not so well protected, it is more vulnerable to injury and other stresses, and its motion is more complicated. Experts caution that, as yet, the artificial knee is not

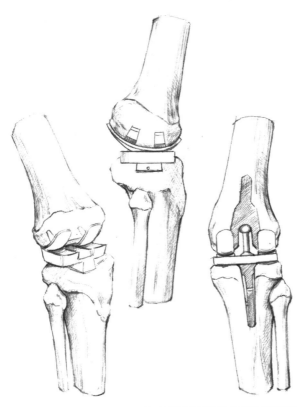

TYPES OF TOTAL KNEE-JOINT REPLACEMENTS.

suitable for patients who are youthfully active and might be inclined to engage in sports. It can be easily damaged by blows as well as by sudden stops and starts.

Probably the first successful device for total knee replacement was developed by the same British group that introduced the successful hip replacement, but many other types that employ a hinge-like mechanism are now being used by European and American surgeons.

The surgery takes from one to two hours or longer. On the average, hospitalization lasts two weeks, with much emphasis on physical therapy to get motion started again. It may take from two to six months before full employment is possible.

The surgeon's fee will probably be about $1,900 to $2,300, the hospitalization about $2,500, and other hospital costs approximately $2,000 to $3,000.

139

Other Replacements

Replacements for other joints are available, but they have not been as successful as those for the hip and the knee. Wrist joint replacements are being inserted with a moderate degree of success, and finger joint replacements have been accomplished by particularly skilled hand surgeons. In the opinion of some experts, however, replacement of finger joints is done more frequently than seems appropriate.

"Many patients with rheumatoid arthritis may have deformed fingers that are not pleasant to look at," says one orthopedist, "but they can do a great deal with those fingers. If you correct the deformity, you may get fingers that look prettier but function worse."

With research in this field of surgery still continuing actively, it is impossible to predict what the future holds. More knowledge is being acquired on how joints function, on how better replacements can be designed, and on how surgical techniques can be improved. Much of this work requires the participation of anatomists, surgeons, mechanical engineers, metallurgists, plastics experts, and even experts who are now investigating new ceramics that represent a spin-off from aerospace research.

The replacement of all the joints, at least in any one patient, does not seem likely, but multiple replacement is already here. For example, one physician with rheumatoid arthritis is alive, well, and practicing medicine while he functions with two total hip replacements, two total knee replacements, two wrist replacements, and an ankle replacement.

CHAPTER 13

"HOW CAN YOU GET THROUGH THE DAY?"

One of the strange facts about arthritis is that some patients with relatively moderate pain and little or no crippling or deformity can be totally devastated emotionally and socially by their illness. In contrast, many with serious disability can have remarkably full, satisfying, useful lives.

Among the latter group, some patients have learned on their own to cope with their arthritis. Others have been helped by their physicians and some by occupational therapists, rehabilitation and vocational counselors, physical therapists, social workers, and nurses—especially visiting nurses—and often by other arthritis patients.

The importance of coping with the psychological and social effects of the disease should not be minimized. "The effects of arthritis can be as disabling to the personality of the arthritic and to his social relationships as they are to his body," one rheumatologist explains. "The outcome of a comprehensive care program for a patient with chronic arthritis may be as dependent on the success of psychological rehabilitation as on the results of medical management."

A woman who had suffered from arthritis for many years put it somewhat differently: "You don't worry about long-term problems," she said. "You try to figure out just one thing—how can you get through the day?"

Often, unfortunately, too little attention is given to this problem. Physicians may be unaware of the nonmedical situation. They may not know how their patients function each day, at home, how they get along with their partners, married or not, or with their children, how they manage to cook or make beds or perform in their jobs. They may not know what fears or frustrations are tormenting their patients. Busy physicians do not normally make house calls and may not have time in an office to ask the proper questions.

And, for whatever reasons, patients don't ask the right questions or openly express their worries and disclose their problems.

All too frequently, patients tell their physicians something less than the whole truth. They do not follow prescribed courses of exercise and rest because they don't see what benefit these could have, or they cannot spare the time from vocational or household responsibilities. They don't take the prescribed drugs because they fail to appreciate their value, but, as one patient put it, "I didn't tell that to my doctor because I didn't want to hurt his feelings."

Often other family members can offer invaluable information to the physician, providing that they have been properly educated on the observations that are critical: changes in the patient's personality, growing depression, more and more frustration, noncompliance with the prescribed treatment, increasing and potentially explosive tensions within the family group. Some of these matters may be alleviated, but only if the physician knows about them. Sometimes the physician should meet privately with the family members, get their views, and perhaps suggest how they can be helpful. A session including physician, patient, and family may have value. Sometimes there is need for a change in the standard treatment program. Sometimes it is obvious that more or less formal psychotherapy must be considered.

If the arthritic disease is no longer in a mild or moderate state but has progressed to a more serious form, it would be remarkable if a patient were *not* beset at least for a while by fears similar to those implied in the following questions:

What are the chances that I will become totally disabled, consigned to a wheelchair or completely bedridden?

The answer now, for all patients with arthritis, is probably about 3 in 100.

What will happen if I can't work? Will I have to spend all my savings and those of my family?

Today about 90 percent or more of all arthritics are employable, although some may need to look for different jobs or job retraining. Referral to a vocational rehabilitation counselor may be of strategic importance. For some patients, unemployability and limited financial resources are very real problems, especially if care from a nonphysician—for example, an occupational therapist—is required, or there is need for a visiting nurse or other home care. Usually such services are not covered by health insurance, although this coverage is now included at least experimentally in a few insurance programs and by some Health Maintenance Organizations, or HMOs. A few governmental programs—notably that of the Veterans Administration—may cover some home services, and the Social Security system is slowly improving its coverage of long-term care. But in too many instances, patients are unable to get this kind of assistance until they have been forced into poverty, and maybe not even then.

How can I make my family and friends realize that I'm not just goofing off and trying to win their pity? How can I make them understand that sometimes I really am exhausted, or depressed, or irritable, or angry, or actually not able to do the tasks that I used to handle?

This one can be a stickler, especially if the patient has few if any visible deformities, and if the other people are themselves healthy. The answer, of course, lies in accurate, adequate knowledge—given to both the patient and the others—about the nature and natural course of the disease, and the effects, desired or undesired, of whatever treatment is applied. Sadly, many health experts may have the needed information but not the time to transmit it to patient and family.

What of the terrible drug side effects that I keep reading about?

The possibility of an adverse drug reaction must never be disregarded. Most such reactions, however, are relatively unimportant and not dangerous. Most serious ones are infrequent. Generally, if there is any untoward reaction—a rash, fever, sore throat, or gastric distress—and this is reported promptly and faithfully to the physician, the problem can be solved by a change in the dosage or the use of a different drug. In many instances, the trouble can be averted if the patient complies precisely with the physician's instructions on the amount and timing of the medication and with directions to get periodic laboratory tests as prescribed. Unfortunately, some patients will, for example, take their medicine between meals when they have been instructed to take it on a full stomach, while others are urged to have a blood test every two weeks but show up for the test every two months.

145

Why do I have all these problems?

It is vital for all patients to recognize that they are not unique, and that other arthritis victims have had to come to grips with these and similar fears. If they cannot obtain adequate reassurance—adequate and honest—from their physicians, other health professionals, or trained social workers, they may be able to get magnificent help and support from other patients. Groups of fellow-sufferers often find it of tremendous help to express their worries openly and hear another member of the group say, for example, "I know what you mean. I went through the same thing myself, and here is what I did . . ." or "Sure, but I got a chance to discuss it with my doctor, and he explained to me that . . ." or "Look, my arthritis has made me more disabled than you, but my husband and I talked it out and we agreed that . . ."

Such group discussions have long since proved their value for people with alcohol or obesity problems, or victims of cancer, or arthritis patients. They are inexpensive, and the main problem is usually getting transportation to the meeting. Church groups, community service organizations, and others dedicated to improving the quality of community life could make an invaluable contribution by organizing them.

Transportation and Other Difficulties

For patients with many chronic diseases, help from physicians and other professionals—physical therapists, nurses, psychologists, social workers, and the like—is available in most cities. In small towns and rural areas, the situation may be more troublesome. For arthritis patients in particular, the key problem may be stated as "But how do I get there?" Many are unable to drive themselves. Bus and streetcar steps are too steep. Transfers are frequently required in public transportation, and these can be a formidable burden. Curbs may represent a menace, and walking even a few blocks can be too painful.

Patients trying to travel on crutches or in a wheelchair may find it impossible to cope with such architectural hor-

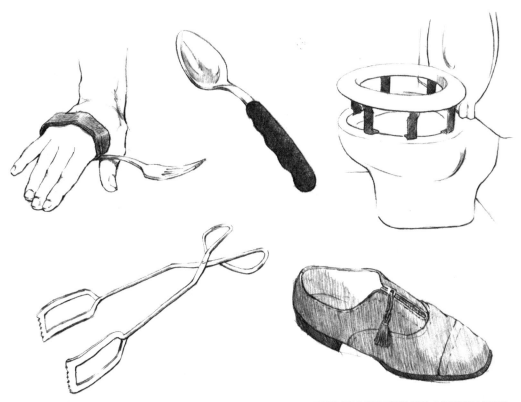

SIMPLE DEVICES HELP PATIENTS DO MANY THINGS WITHOUT ASSISTANCE.

rors as narrow doorways to toilets or telephone booths, or restrooms that can be reached only via a flight of steps. This stair problem may be found in many restaurants and theaters, both old and new. Ironically, to our own knowledge, it may be found in at least one medico-dental building where patients are supposed to come and see their physicians.

More and more, governmental agencies and private groups are recognizing the existence of such problems for the disabled. Some are organizing low-cost or free transportation services from home to hospital or physician's office. They are including ramps along the steps at the entrance to buildings. They are cutting ramps into sidewalks at each street corner, so designed that they can be navigated by someone in a wheelchair.

In the same way, ingenious and often inexpensive modifications can be made in the patient's home—installing railings wherever they are needed to provide support, building ramps, raising the height of toilet seats, and providing

147

easier-to-reach storage areas in kitchens. Numerous devices can now be purchased to enable patients to protect the joints that are painful and disabled while making better use of the joints that are undamaged—gadgets for opening cans, for putting on and removing shoes, for getting into and out of chairs, for assistance in walking, coping with zippers, for holding a telephone.*

Here, too, patients conferring in groups can offer or acquire useful suggestions. "Let me tell you how I learned to open and close a car door," or "If you have such trouble getting the coffee from the top shelf, why do you put it there in the first place?" or "If you can't manage a heavy soup pot, divide the soup in half and cook it in two small pots," or "Forget how it may look to your relatives. If it makes you a little less dependent, do it!"

In professional circles, such matters are in the province of what is termed occupational therapy. Some medical centers are well-staffed with trained, competent occupational therapists. Others, including several that depict themselves as demonstration centers for the very best in health care, are woefully deficient.

One reason for various deficiencies in the care of arthritis patients has been the very nature of medical education. Until perhaps five or ten years ago, most so-called modern medical training was essentially crisis-oriented and hospital-based. (In some teaching institutions, it still is.) Students had their attention focused on the dramatic heart attack, the brain concussion, the acute appendicitis, or the life-threatening hemorrhage or blood clot. With few exceptions, medical students learned relatively little about chronic illness, only to discover when they began their practices outside of a hospital that *many* of their patients were suffering from chronic disease. Only then did they learn that the care of chronic disease patients is usually undramatic, unexciting, exceedingly difficult—sometimes far more difficult than attending to a crisis.

In recent years, many and perhaps most medical schools have changed their approach. They are now graduating young physicians who are increasingly aware of the chronic disease problem. They know how to help chronically ill pa-

* For a catalog of such devices, see the list of suggested references on page 195.

tients and understand the need for long-term care. Particularly important are the new three-year postgraduate residencies in family practice that are now being developed in many parts of the United States.

The training of other health professionals—physical therapists, occupational therapists, and others—could undoubtedly be improved by a similar modernization, enabling them to provide even more help to patients with arthritis and other chronic illnesses.

A second problem comes from the all too evident fact that long-term care is long term. Treatment over a period of years—sometimes for many years—may be needed. And, with shockingly few exceptions, the United States has yet to find satisfactory ways to finance this kind of care. Most governmental and third-party health insurance programs include only limited coverage for health care that is not hospital-based or delivered by a physician. Yet there is abundant evidence that outpatient physical therapy, vocational counseling, and other outpatient health services can do much to keep arthritis patients employable and off the welfare rolls, but the costs may be more than most patients can afford.

CHAPTER 14

ARTHRITIS
AND SEXUALITY

Since the early reports of Kinsey and Masters and Johnson, there has been growing interest in sex and sexuality and a willingness to discuss sexual concerns openly. These concerns may occur in anyone, healthy or ill. They may be particularly serious in victims of arthritis whose problems are often intensified by pain, crippling, difficulties in motion, deformity, and frustration.

At the base of such concerns is the widespread belief that the only goal of sexuality is sexual intercourse. Instead, as experienced sex counselors emphasize, the goal is the expression of love and affection and satisfactory communication.

Because of the growing recognition of this desired end, and because many physicians feel they are not adequately knowledgeable or are embarrassed to discuss the subject, special sex counselors are now being used to work with arthritis patients and victims of other chronic diseases.

The Kinds of Help

Probably the first need of a concerned patient is to be able to talk with his or her partner, if there is one. Perhaps there is a need to communicate first with somebody else. (The primary need is not simply to be told of alternative positions, or exercises to be tried and practiced.)

Effective sex counselors find they can be most helpful at the outset if they can give "permission" to the patient to communicate—for the patient to say, for example, "Intercourse isn't actually that vital to me. I'd know he loves me if he touches me, or kisses me, or caresses me," or "There are other ways she can give me pleasure, but I'm afraid to men-

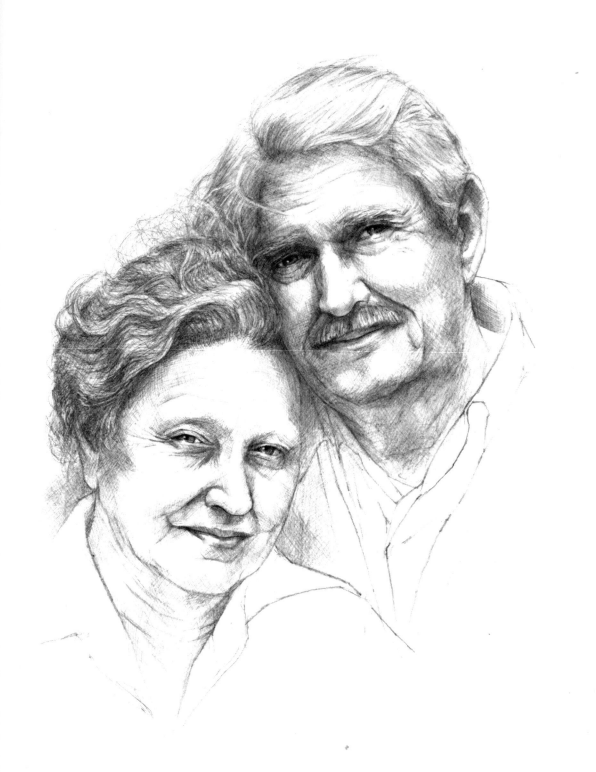

tion them to her," or "What I really want is some sign that he needs me," or "With my twisted, deformed fingers, I'm sure he thinks I'm ugly."

One experienced counselor says, "We can let patients find that there are lots of ways to be sexual, and these aren't second-class ways, either. We can help them find ways that will fit each person or each couple."

How does such a couple find the way that will fit? At the outset, by discussion—learning, perhaps for the first time, what each likes, what each doesn't like, what each transmits, receives, and interprets as a signal of love. Counselors emphasize that this learning process may not be a once-in-a-lifetime procedure. As people get older, likes and dislikes may change. If arthritis strikes, they almost certainly will change, but the individuals can learn to adjust accordingly.

With exceedingly few if any exceptions, arthritis patients and their partners must be aware that no sexual activity can make the arthritic disease worse. Likewise, they must be aware that the patient may occasionally go through a period of depression and may not have any interest in sexuality, affection, or virtually anything else, but these periods generally pass.

The Sources of Help

Some physicians believe they are competent to provide all the information on sexuality that patients may require. Others do not hold such an idea. Most, it appears, rarely mention the subject while asking probing questions about virtually every other aspect of the patient's life. If the patient brings up the subject, the physician may be embarrassed.

One result of these divergent views was indicated in a recent study of a large number of family practitioners and internists. One group reported that less than 4 percent of their patients had any concerns about sexuality, while another group declared that such concerns affected 20 to 30 percent of their patients. It was the second group that felt reasonably comfortable in talking about sexuality and often brought up the subject themselves. Sexuality researchers put the figure as high as 80 percent, ranging all the way from trivial concerns at one end of the scale to major sex problems at the other.

Among the various health professionals, the most helpful—whether it be physician, nurse, psychologist, marriage relations counselor, occupational counselor, or sex counselor—is the one who is both knowledgeable and able to discuss sexuality concerns with complete comfort.

Some patients, and perhaps many of them, need little or no help from professionals. Excellent books are now readily available, and often they can provide the necessary help.* Others can receive substantial assistance from a few brief sessions with a counselor, possibly for an hour or two. Occasionally, patients say, all they need is a few minutes to sit down and talk to someone who doesn't make judgments or offer sure cures. Rarely, it appears, is there a need for full-scale psychotherapy.

In many of these different approaches, the patient or the couple may work alone with one sex counselor. Sometimes it is more helpful if two counselors take part. Often group sessions are productive—and generally less expensive. In no case should the partner be an unwilling participant in the treatment. "If the partner has to be dragged in," an expert says, "everybody is just wasting time." It must also be recognized that some individuals, for whatever reasons, are not candidates for help; they are not and apparently cannot be made comfortable in talking about sexuality, and they refuse to answer any questions on the subject. If the subject is raised, the situation may be made worse.

In our own medical center, the University of California, San Francisco, many of us have been interested in a long-term demonstration project supported by the National Institute for Mental Health, aimed at training counselors to cope with a variety of sexuality concerns in patients with arthritis and other chronic illnesses. The students—many of them with physical limitations themselves—have come from all parts of the United States to undergo training that takes twenty hours a week for a full year. They have so far included people who already have had formal training in rehabilitation, social welfare, psychology, and similar fields, or who have long been active in the community to help disabled men and women. Plans are underway to have such a counselor assigned regularly to our arthritis clinic.

This training program is probably the first of its kind in

* See the section at the end of this book on suggested references.

the United States. Almost all major medical centers, however, maintain their own counseling services or can refer patients to such services elsewhere.

Referral from this kind of a center can usually mean assurance that the patient will be sent to a trained professional. In California and many other states, such professionals as psychologists, marriage counselors, occupational therapists, and social workers are licensed by the state and required to take both formal courses and in-service training, sometimes for several thousand hours. On the other hand, virtually anyone can take a week-end seminar and then hang up a shingle proclaiming himself or herself to be an sex expert.

The important point is this: with or without professional help, there can be a satisfying expression of love, affection, and sexuality—even with arthritis.

CHAPTER 15

THE ARTHRITIS TEAM

As is true of many other chronic illnesses, arthritis in its severe forms can cause problems so complex, so interwoven, and so difficult that few if any health professionals can by themselves help the patient to cope with them. In such instances, the mobilization of a team of experts may be desirable or even essential.

In this chapter, the responsibilities of these experts are presented. It is uncommon for the expertise of all of them to be required for an individual case. Often, one professional can do double duty: a visiting nurse, for example, can teach the patient how to follow a prescribed physical therapy program. A pharmacist can not merely dispense a drug, but also reinforce the physician's instructions on how to use it. Virtually all of these professionals can help by educating patients and family members.

Whatever the membership of the arthritis team, the first question is who should run it. Or, in other words, how does the patient find—and keep—the right doctor?

The Physician

Some years ago, several of our medical friends, together with a remarkable public relations executive, outlined a new prescription. It was designed to alleviate a lot of what had gone wrong with patient-physician relationships.

Every patient, the proposal declared, should have his or her own personal physician, one who would speak for all the components of medicine *to* the patient and *for* the patient to all of medicine.

If, for example, a patient awoke in the middle of the night with severe abdominal pain, he would not attempt to

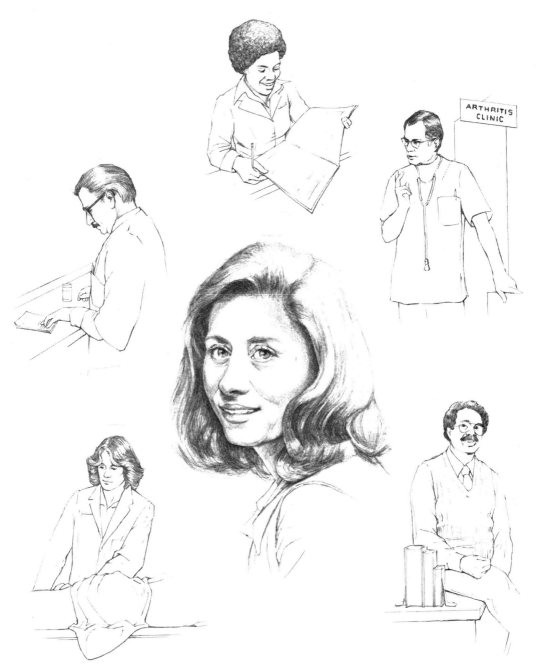

THE ARTHRITIS TEAM.

decide whether to call an internist, an abdominal surgeon, a stomach specialist, or a psychiatrist. He should call his personal physician. If that physician could handle the problem himself, he would do so. If he couldn't determine the cause or the treatment, he should say so at once without any loss of face and suggest summoning the appropriate specialist.

Never, however, should the personal physician refer the patient to somebody else and then drop out of the picture, a procedure that almost always transforms a human being into Case No. 1,234 or "the fascinating hernia in Room 567." Rather, the specialist should be asked to join the group, while the personal physician would visit the patient in the hospital, if necessary, and follow every development. The personal physician must be responsible for explaining what is being done—in case the specialist is too busy or unable to speak intelligibly. If the specialist is not doing a good job, the patient should not be put through the embarrassment of discharging him. The personal physician should shoulder that responsibility.

The particular specialty of the personal physician may not be particularly important. He may be a family practitioner, an internist, a pediatrician, or a surgeon. Or even a specialist in rheumatology. Other matters are far more essential:

The patient must like and respect the physician as a specially skilled but not perfect human being.

The patient must not expect the physician to know all the answers, and he must value the physician's honest admission that he is baffled and wants expert assistance.

The physician must like and respect the patient as a human being. In addition, the physician must get to know the patient's fears and hopes, his family structure and the strengths and weaknesses of that structure, the nature of his job, his financial resources, his diet, his drinking habits, and his pattern of self-medication.

Just as the patient must realize that time is money for the physician, and that some prolonged stays in waiting rooms are inevitable, the physician must realize that time may also represent money for the patient.

The patient must understand that no diagnostic procedure or treatment is foolproof; nor can it be guaranteed to give the hoped-for outcome in every case. An outcome that is not completely satisfactory or an adverse reaction is not necessarily evidence of negligence.

163

Is it difficult to develop such a physician-patient relationship? It most certainly is difficult and time-consuming, and it can rarely be done in a few office visits. In some depersonalized health care programs, it may be impossible. But when this relationship can be achieved, it can be invaluable.

The physician should properly be the captain of the arthritis team; but, as one critic declared a few years ago, he must not think that he owns the team. If he is well-trained, experienced, competent, compassionate, sensitive, and willing to accept his own limitations, the team will generally function well. And the patient will benefit.

For the majority of arthritis patients, the physician will be in family practice, an internist (one who specializes in internal medicine), or a pediatrician. Chances are that a family practitioner or internist will already know the patient and the other family members, having treated them for a variety of ills.

In relatively few cases, a rheumatologist will be called on for consultation. There are believed to be only about three thousand such experts in the United States, and their geographic distribution is not uniform. Some states may have only one or two. Some may have none.

When surgery is needed, consultation may be sought from an orthopedic surgeon, rather than a general surgeon, and especially an orthopedist who has had long experience in performing arthritis surgery. Like rheumatologists, orthopedic surgeons competent to handle such procedures as a total knee replacement are few in number and unequally distributed. Most practice only in or near major medical centers because of the need for special facilities and surgical teams experienced in working together.

For patients living in small cities or rural areas, obtaining access to specialists like these may pose a serious problem. As emphasized earlier, a team approach will often be required during convalescence after major joint surgery.

Nursing Care

In the hospital, the nurse may take an active and important part in arthritis treatment. Perhaps an even more strategic role can be played by the public health nurse or visiting nurse who sees the patient at home. Such a professional can inform the physician about the patient's home environment and physical and emotional problems, needs, fears, and aspirations. At the same time, the nurse can reinforce or clarify the physician's explanations and directions, teaching the patient how to perform exercises, apply hot or cold compresses, follow dietary advice, and use splints, crutches, and other devices. Often the visiting nurse will find that, regardless of what the physician is told, the patient is not taking drugs or following recommended exercises as prescribed.

As the arthritic disease becomes better or worse, it is often the nurse who can best suggest to the physician changes in the treatment program and who can help the patient maintain the necessary physical, mental, and social equilibrium.

In many cases in which other family members have not been appropriately briefed on the situation, it is the visiting nurse who can supply the essential information. Often, the nurse is the first to recognize that other members of the arthritis health team should be mobilized.

Occupational Therapy

When one or more joints are seriously damaged by arthritis, it is often the occupational therapist who can best help the patient make optimum use of the remaining healthy joints in order to perform the routine tasks of daily living. Through formal training and practical experience, such therapists can demonstrate new and painless ways to dress and undress, clean, make beds, cook, utilize storage space efficiently, handle tools, drive a car, and the like. They can recommend devices and gadgets that can be built or purchased. If there is severe pain in foot joints, the therapist may suggest the use of special shoes. Consultation with a podiatrist may be helpful.

If the physician is unable to recommend a competent occupational therapist, most hospitals maintain lists of available experts, and many have one or more such therapists on the hospital staff.

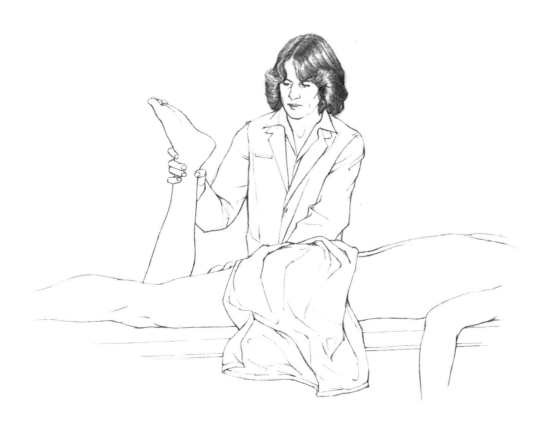

Physical Therapy

As with nursing care, physical therapy may be provided in the hospital, but most often it is applied in the therapist's office. Here the goals are to have the patients learn how to stand, walk, and sit properly, and even how to lie in bed properly, to teach them how to maintain or improve muscle and joint function by appropriate exercises, how to breathe properly, and how to use heat or cold applications (primarily to enable them to exercise with a minimum of pain). In some cases, it is necessary to show family members how to assist patients in performing the exercises.

As with nursing and the provision of other professional services, the physical therapy program is either directed by the physician or laid out in consultation between physician and physical therapist. Usually the patient will need to see a physical therapist only a few times at the outset and then once every several weeks or even less frequently.

Orthotics

Often it is desirable to protect a painful joint by the use of a special brace or splint. These supports are not the heavy plaster casts used, for example, to immobilize a broken arm or leg. Most of the orthopedic appliances employed in arthritis treatment are made of a lightweight plastic or metal, and are usually worn only at night or for a few hours during the day. Frequently, they are molded specifically to fit an individual patient.

Working under the direction of the physician, an orthotist—the new name for this kind of specialist—may also design special shoes and other foot supports.

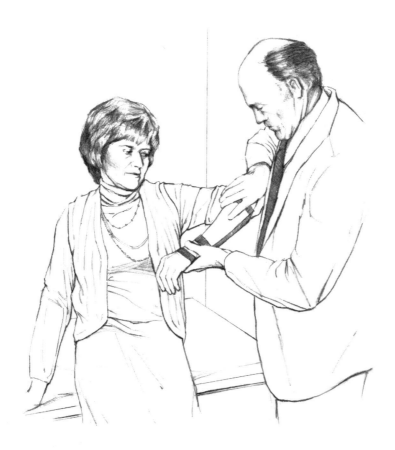

Pharmacy

Currently, there are some six thousand different prescription drugs on the market, and no physician can keep up with all or even many of them. But this is the pharmacist's major specialty. Accordingly, physicians—except for some specialists—are frequently turning to pharmacists for advice and consultation. After the diagnosis has been established and the general course of treatment outlined, the physician may consult with the pharmacist to select the particular product and dosage to be prescribed for a particular patient, and the drugs *not* to be prescribed, and to indicate which drugs are most likely to interact dangerously with which other prescription or over-the-counter products.

In the specific case of arthritis, it is probable that pharmacists see more victims of the disease than do physicians, and almost certainly the pharmacists see them earlier in the course of their disease. They can often spot self-treating people who are repeatedly trying one over-the-counter painkiller after another in order to relieve arthritis symptoms and can urge those people to seek medical care. In some cases, the pharmacist knows that the patient is also taking other remedies—prescription or over-the-counter—that may interact with the antiarthritis drug (patients sometimes forget to mention other drugs to their physicians). Occasionally, the pharmacist can suggest ways to reduce drug costs, especially when inexpensive generic-name products are available. And often it is the pharmacist who is the first to be aware that an arthritis patient has forgotten or neglected to get a refill of a prescription and can relay this information to the physician.

Where it is possible, many patients or families can benefit from having a personal or family pharmacist.

Psychotherapy

Although most patients with arthritis probably do not need psychiatric help, there is a distinct psychosocial component in many forms of the disease. The problems may well be discussed with the patient's own physician. Depending on the circumstances, it may be helpful for the patient to have an opportunity to discuss emotional problems with a psychiatrist. In those instances in which psychotherapy is indicated, patients may benefit significantly. In some cases, the patient may elect to enter therapy with a clinical psychologist rather than a psychiatrist.

Nutrition

For the many arthritis patients who are seriously overweight or using deficient diets, a dietician may contribute significantly by recommending a reducing diet or one that contains the appropriate quantities of essential food elements. Reducing diets may be particularly important for some patients about to undergo joint surgery.

Vocational Rehabilitation

Vocational rehabilitation is aimed at finding jobs for which disabled patients are employable or retraining them so they can be employable. This form of counselling is now supported by federal funds, but it is not used adequately for those with arthritis and other chronic illnesses. Critics have charged that the system is governed not by medical needs but by impersonal economics. It is too often hampered by bureaucratic regulations and practices. Communications with potential employers are inadequate. Patients with possibly increasing disability are viewed pessimistically. And perhaps most unfortunately, many physicians and other health professionals fail to refer an arthritis patient to a rehabilitation counselor.

Social Work

Ideally, the social worker as a member of the health team can serve as ombudsperson, coordinator, patient advocate, and guide for both patient and physician through the bewildering maze of governmental and institutional red tape, regulations, wildly inconsistent eligibility rules, overlapping requirements, and—all too often—inadequate funds.

Visiting a patient's home, a competent social worker need not have much detailed knowledge about arthritis but can discover a great deal about the patient and the family— their needs, problems, goals, and resources. Often such a worker can be the first to spot growing tensions within the family group. Many social workers have had substantial training in helping patients cope with psychological problems, and with such physical problems as inadequate living conditions. Usually the experienced worker will know more about the availability of such services as "meals on wheels" and other needed facilities and resources in the community than will any other health team member.

Social workers and other members of the team can help to initiate and organize group sessions in which arthritis patients can help each other to cope with a wide range of social, psychological, physical, and vocational problems. In the case of a severely disabled victim who has required fulltime care, month after month, from a son and daughter-in-law, for example, they can attempt to arrange temporary live-in help for perhaps two weeks in order to give the younger people at least a brief respite. Or, as has been done in some European countries, they can arrange for a short-term nursing home or hospital stay for the patient while the others get a vacation break.

The composition and the activities of the arthritis health team may be drastically limited by the patient's health insurance coverage and financial assets.

Under most governmental and private third-party health programs, coverage of physician and hospital bills is substantial. So is coverage of nursing, physical therapy and similar services, but only if they are provided to hospitalized patients. Few of these programs offer significant help to patients after they leave the hospital and may require long-term care extending over years and possibly a lifetime. The financial problem is particularly serious for those who need long-term care from health professionals who are not physicians. It is encouraging, however, to note that some health maintenance organizations and prepaid health plans are providing for substantial home-care services, not only because they are medically indicated, but because in the long run they save money for the program.

Unlike other countries which have attempted to find solutions for this vexing question, the United States so far has done exceedingly little. As a nation, we have not yet faced up to the issue. It is time that we come to grips with it.

CHAPTER 16

ACUPUNCTURE, HYPNOSIS, AND MANIPULATION

Especially since the early 1970s, there has been considerable interest in the value of acupuncture to control or even cure a wide variety of diseases. Used in China and other countries for thousands of years, the technique consists of placing special needles in carefully designated parts of the body, particularly to control pain.

Many practitioners—physicians and nonphysicians alike—in the United States and Europe have attempted to evaluate acupuncture in the control of arthritis, along with the claims that range from brilliant success to total failure. At the University of California medical center in San Francisco, trials on patients by experienced acupuncturists have produced the conclusion that the procedure has little value in treating rheumatoid arthritis. There seems to be temporary relief of pain for some, but the treatment has no significant effect on the underlying inflammation and the progression of the disease.

Some observers have expressed the view that acupuncture is, in fact, a form of hypnotism, and medical hypnotists have attempted to use hypnotherapy on arthritis patients. In some cases, hypnotism has apparently lessened pain temporarily and possibly improved mobility, but the progress of the disease has not been affected.

A patient who has one of the many common forms of arthritis may turn to manipulation of the spine—most often by a chiropractor—to correct what may be or merely be thought to be a misalignment of the vertebrae, causing pressure on spinal nerves. There may not be one bit of x-ray evidence to show the existence of any such vertebral displacement; nevertheless, the patient may be subjected to a variety of manipulative procedures—kneading, pulling, twisting, stretching, jerking, and the like.

175

Usually, patients seeking this kind of treatment are those who either have no faith in physicians or surgeons in the first place or are disappointed with the failure of any medical treatment to produce prompt improvement.

In some cases, the manipulation is temporarily beneficial. In general, the happy results are the ones most likely to be reported to friends and relatives and particularly other patients, occasionally in the form of a signed testimonial. But, when the maneuvers yield no lasting help or result in injury, patients are less likely to publicize the fact. Furthermore, a patient may spend hundreds or thousands of dollars for manipulation before seeking medical or surgical help.

Tragically, especially in rheumatoid arthritis, careless manipulation of the vertebrae—whether performed by a physician, a physical therapist, or a chiropractor—can cause the rupture of a vertebral disc or the fracture of one or more vertebrae. It can result in permanent nerve injury. In some cases, overly vigorous manipulation of the neck can damage or even sever the spinal cord, causing permanent paralysis or death.

Most authorities are in agreement that manipulative procedures are infrequently beneficial and all too frequently represent unnecessary expenditures.

CHAPTER 17

THE SPECIAL
ARTHRITIS DIET

Forget it. There isn't any.

There is no scientific evidence that arthritis can be helped or worsened by any vitamin, mineral, protein, fat, or carbohydrate. If patients decide to embark on a diet of yoghurt, organic foods, vegetable juice, alkaline foods, or acid foods, it probably won't hurt them.

Previous generations of physicians were accustomed to advising patients with gout to avoid "rich" or "high purine" foods—sweetbreads, kidneys, liver, goose, and the like. With the advent of the new antigout remedies, the control of the disease is usually so simple that it is rarely necessary to lay down strict dietary restrictions.

In the case of alcoholic beverages, some physicians recommend complete abstinence in gout. Others feel that alcohol in moderation is permissible. It is difficult to speak out against moderate drinking.

For one whose weight-bearing joints—those in the feet, knees, and hips—were designed to support a body weight of perhaps 150 pounds, a weight of 200 pounds or more can do no good and may contribute to joint damage. In such a case, weight control through diet may be required.

Otherwise, for arthritis patients, eat and enjoy. *Bon appetit!*

CHAPTER 18

QUACKERY

[*The Arthritis Goldmine*]

It is in the nature of arthritis and many other conditions—asthma, multiple sclerosis, epilepsy, and some forms of cancer—that there are good days and there are bad days. Inexplicably, the disease goes through occasional but unpredictable ups and downs. Sometimes, regardless of which treatment is given or not given, the patient feels better. At other times, the patient feels worse.

Few aspects of chronic disease are so puzzling, and few have been more profitable for the purveyors of nostrums and quack remedies. Estimates of the amount wasted on these each year for arthritis alone run to $485 million.

If the improvement happens to coincide with ingestion of, say, Vitamin E, or with the commencement of a diet of organic foods, it is understandable that it will be attributed to the offbeat remedy. It is likewise understandable that the happy patient will pass on the news to friends, and a miraculous new "cure" myth will have been born. It has been noted, however, that, when the newly discovered remedy no longer works and the symptoms return, the patient is less eager to mention this to friends. Meanwhile, the news of the discovery may have already been enshrined in a television report, a newspaper story, a magazine article, or a book.

In the past, the unproved remedies proposed and actually used on arthritis victims have ranged from the harmless but nonsensical to the dangerous and potentially lethal.

183

Included in the list are these:

> Liver juice and cod liver oil (to lubricate the joints)
> Multivitamins
> Vitamin E in particular (this one was introduced when cortisone—known in the early days as Compound E—was expensive and in short supply, and some enterprising people convinced many patients that Vitamin E was the same thing)
> Honey and vinegar
> Herbal treatments
> Mineral waters
> Bee venom
> Cobra venom
> Flushing out the colon
> Sulfur baths
> Bleedings
> Application of a hot poker
> Fasting
> Injecting distilled water into the hip
> Carrying a talisman or an apple in the hip pocket
> Electric shocks
> Sitting for prolonged periods in an abandoned uranium mine
> Wearing certain jewelry, such as copper bracelets
> Eating only uncooked foods
> Eating only cooked foods

Protagonists of these and similar treatments (who have sometimes profited handsomely from them) usually say that their ideas have not been accepted by most scientists and physicians because of some "conspiracy" in the scientific-medical establishment. It should be noted here that scientists and physicians and members of their families also suffer from arthritis and would relish the discovery of agents more useful than those now accepted.

One of the most serious forms of what should be considered quackery is the use of generally accepted drugs in incredibly large doses or for incredibly long periods. These treatments, widely promoted and costly, have been administered particularly in a few Mexican clinics, to the distress of distinguished Mexican rheumatologists. The drugs usually employed are phenylbutazone or one of its derivatives and one or more of the adrenal corticosteroid hormones. Each can produce serious tissue damage or death.

Over many decades, the press has carried glowing accounts of patients who returned after their treatment in the Mexican clinics with their pain relieved, their stiffness lessened, and their joyous euphoria a delight to behold. Less attention was paid to what happened later—the damage to blood-forming organs, the bone-softening, the fractured vertebrae, the psychotic changes, and, in some cases, the deaths. Among the victims were patients who went to Mexico for treatment and then returned home with a large supply— perhaps 500 tablets or more—of high-dosage corticosteroid hormones, along with instructions to return just before the supply runs out to get a refill. A number of the patients felt so much improved and so euphoric by the therapy that they decided the problem had been solved and there was no need to obtain more of the medication. They soon discovered what most physicians have long known: sudden termination of high-dosage steroid treatment can have catastrophic effects. Unfortunately, the accounts of these and other misadventures have generally been restricted to medical journals and autopsy reports.

Patients curious about any antiarthritis "cure" can usually get information promptly from the Arthritis Foundation* or the National Institute of Arthritis, Metabolism and Digestive Diseases.†

---

* Arthritis Foundation, Lenox P.O. Box 18,888, Atlanta GA 30326
† National Institute of Arthritis, Metabolism and Digestive Diseases, Bethesda MD 20014

CHAPTER 19

THE
ARTHRITIS PLAN

Most arthritis patients will generally need only occasional medical treatment. But millions of others can benefit greatly from high-quality, properly organized long-term care. Such care should be based on out-of-hospital programs. It should be aimed at maintaining maximum freedom from dependency on others and at allowing patients to live in a normal environment as long as possible.

The details of this kind of approach have already been blueprinted. No revolutionary new discoveries are required. Sadly, however, the needed services are often located too far away or are too costly. Patients—and many such primary care physicians as family doctors, internists, and pediatricians—may not even be aware of them.

The results: pain that could have been alleviated, crippling and deformity that could have been prevented or corrected, unemployability that need not have occurred.

A most significant step to correct this unhappy state of affairs came in 1975 with the passage of the National Arthritis Act, a signal that, for the first time in history, the Congress and the President recognized the seriousness of the arthritis problem. As a result of this legislation, a national commission of arthritis experts and members of the general public (including several arthritis patients) conducted nationwide hearings, conferences, and investigations. In 1976, the commission submitted to the Congress its recommendations for action. Those recommendations are generally known now as the National Arthritis Plan. The major goals are:

Every American should be aware of the early symptoms of the most common forms of arthritis and recognize the need to seek professional care.

Every family physician, internist, and pediatrician should be aware of the basic techniques for arthritis diagnosis and treatment, and know when and where to refer patients for specialized care.

Teaching programs in arthritis should exist in every medical school. (Most schools allot only a few hours of the curriculum to the study of arthritis, and about one-tenth have no special faculty or specific program in rheumatology.)

Research efforts should be greatly intensified.

Arthritis centers or community programs should be accessible to major population areas.

In general, the arthritis community programs should be designed and developed so that they can serve as models for nationwide action against other chronic disease.

A keystone of the Arthritis Plan is the creation of multipurpose arthritis centers in teaching institutions around the country. As defined in the Plan, each is not to be a structure of steel and concrete, but rather a group of cooperating health professionals. In each case, the program and facilities must be designed to demonstrate and stimulate the prompt and effective application of knowledge already available, and to develop urgently needed new knowledge. More than twenty of these centers have already been approved, with funds available for their operation.

Of the many possible center activities, the highest priority is to be given the training of every needed variety of health professional. Such people are needed not only to provide health care and to train other professionals, but also to help guide patients through the current maze of services that may include different health specialists, different state and federal agencies, different eligibility requirements, and different insurance or third-party programs. The chronically ill patient with arthritis is probably the least able to find the way through what is now an almost unbelievable labyrinth.

Almost as much emphasis is to be put on the development of community programs through which satellite clinics, mobile units, and other systems will be employed to demonstrate throughout the community the best possible long-term care of arthritis.

Throughout, heavy emphasis must be placed on research. With a few important exceptions, as already noted, there is no treatment now that will truly cure arthritis. A major reason is that, again with few exceptions, the cause of arthritis is unknown.

Much of this shortage of knowledge can be blamed on the lack of funds. In fiscal year 1978–79, for example, the National Institutes of Health—probably the largest research organization in the world—are scheduled to spend about $50 million for arthritis research and related activities. Of this sum, roughly $35 million is earmarked for the National Institute of Arthritis, Metabolism and Digestive Diseases. The $50 million equals roughly $1.61 for each arthritis patient in the United States. In striking contrast, $508 million is planned for the National Heart, Lung and Blood Institute and $937 million for the National Cancer Institute.

In the United States, it has been said that our standard procedure for solving any problem is to throw money at it. Such a solution has obviously not been attempted in the case of arthritis.

Recent discoveries in the field of arthritis warrant heavy support for research. The most exciting among them is the finding that there is now almost indisputable evidence of an inherited susceptibility to some forms of the disease. There is also increasing evidence that, in other forms, an immune mechanism plays a part. In addition, improved joint replacements should be designed and new classes of potential drugs call for investigation.

Building on clues like these, research workers are becoming increasingly confident that they can unravel the factors that cause arthritis, and perhaps find practical methods to prevent it.

Obviously, the eventual conquest of arthritis is not around the corner. On the other hand, it may not be as far away as we once thought.

SUGGESTED
REFERENCES

Allied Health Professions Section, The Arthritis Foundation, *Self-Help Manual for Arthritis Patients* (Atlanta, Georgia: The Arthritis Foundation). (This book describes many devices for self-help and indicates where they may be obtained.)

Barbach, Lonnie Garfield, *For Yourself: The Fulfillment of Female Sexuality* (New York: Doubleday, 1975).

Calabro, John J., and Wykert, John, *The Truth About Arthritis Care* (New York: David McKay, 1971).

Crain, Darrell C., *The Arthritis Handbook: A Patient's Manual on Arthritis and Rheumatism and Gout*, 2d ed. (New York: Arco, 1971).

Zilbergeld, Bernie, *Male Sexuality* (Boston: Little, Brown, 1978).

The following pamphlets can be obtained from The Arthritis Foundation, 3400 Peachtree Road, N.E., Atlanta, Georgia 30326, or from local chapters of the Foundation.

Arthritis: The Basic Facts
Rheumatoid Arthritis: A Handbook for Patients
Osteoarthritis: A Handbook for Patients
Home Care Programs in Arthritis: A Manual for Patients
Living with Arthritis
About Gout
SLE: Systemic Lupus Erythematosus

INDEX